SARINA WHEATMAN

Communication and Connection

(AKA - Relapse Prevention)

Michael Terence Publishing

First published in paperback by
Michael Terence Publishing in 2022
www.mtp.agency

ISBN 9781800943520

This book is dedicated to all the people past and present who have Contributed by trying, some succeeding and some still struggling To walk the recovery road with me.

You have all taught me much that has helped me better understand this illness.

To my brilliant and strong, much missed mother who Taught me to be curious and never give up.

To Olivia de Gruchey, soul sister, walker of the 12-step way.

I miss your wisdom every single day.

Contents

About Sarina Wheatman

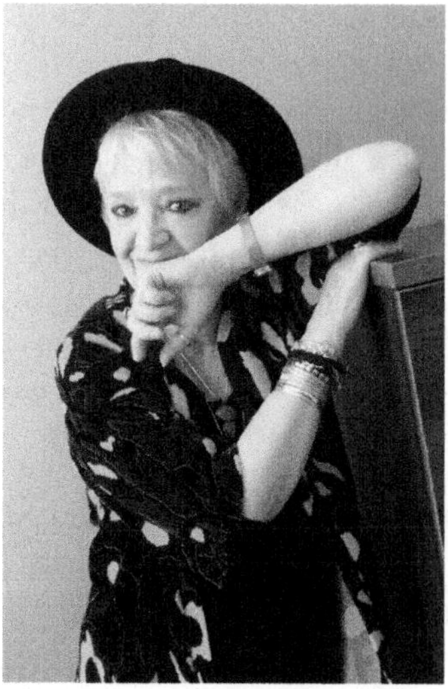

Addiction has been a very strange phenomenon in my life, first of all when I was pretty young it tried to convince me it was cool and the only way to live, whilst at the same time eroding any value system I had. As the disease progressed in me I began to realise it was creating in me a person I did not like or want to be. It was also trying to kill me. I, thank goodness found my way out of the maze that addiction creates and became well.

Needing to leave a hedonistic lifestyle behind where, new people and new countries and new jobs were my way of coping with my deteriorating behaviour I discovered something that caught my attention. Recovery, first of all for myself, and later when I had become more stable and able to be more the version of me I was supposed to be, I started to train as a therapist.

This journey of recovery has taken thirty-eight years, full of ups and downs, twists, and turns. At the moment I live and work in the South of England, I work in a rehab, I also have a small private practice. My love of writing happened late in my life. I disliked school with a vengeance and left at the earliest opportunity, but my chosen career made it possible to go back to study in college, where to my surprise I found I loved studying and homework and researching. My passion for all things recovery has made me desire to be able to change perceptions about addiction, and to make recovery more accessible for more people, hence the books.

Today I live and work and write about addiction and recovery. So addiction is a very strange phenomenon indeed, which most people who are lucky enough to find recovery will attest to. First a destroyer of all values and potential killer, and then a twist of fate and the knowledge of it can be used for the greater good.

Mental Wellness is defined by the World Health Organisation as:

"A state of well-being in which the individual realises his or her own abilities, can cope with the normal stresses of life, can work productively and fruitfully, and is able to make a contribution to his or her community.

Mental wellness is more than just the absence of mental illness."

Foreword

I am a registered Medical Doctor and was appointed to my first Consultant role as a General Adult Psychiatrist in Southampton in 1999. I work as the Consultant Lead in General Adult and Addiction Psychiatry at The Manor Clinic, Southampton, a residential facility for management of Alcohol and Substance Dependence. I have worked as a Consultant Psychiatrist in General Adult Psychiatry, both within the NHS and Independent Sectors.

I trained in General Adult Psychiatry at the Maudsley Hospital, London; The Institute of Psychiatry, Psychology and Neuroscience (loPPN - Kings College London), and in Liaison Psychiatry at Kings College Hospital, London. I trained in Addiction Psychiatry on the National Addiction unit – The Maudsley Hospital; and in neuropsychiatric disorders such as Attention Deficit Hyperactive Disorder (ADHD). I have been a Member of The Royal College of Psychiatrists since 1996 and elected a Fellow in 2018.

I first met Sarina, when we worked together at the Priory Hospital Southampton, in 2001 when Sarina was the Lead Therapist on the Eating Disorder Service. She was already an outstanding Therapist in Eating Disorders and Chemical and Behavioural addictions. She has been in recovery from addiction for the past 30 years. It has been a pleasure to work with her again when I came to The Manor Clinic on a regular basis in 2017. The Clinic has been changing lives and helping people to start their recovery journeys since 2006.

Sarina has made her own remarkable journey from her individual recovery from addiction; via AA; personal therapy and then her training as a therapist. She describes that this process 'saved her life'. What is equally remarkable is the manner in which she has dedicated her professional and personal life to help others overcome addiction. During her journey as a therapist, lead therapist in Eating Disorder Services and addiction services she has worked with countless individuals, and their families to help them navigate their own journey to recovery and freedom from addiction.

I've also witnessed her migrate from helping individuals and their families, to helping disseminate the principals of 'Recovery from Addiction' in her writings and books. To be able to distil the essentials of recovery and communicate them to others through her writing is a rare gift. She continually strives to understand mental health illness's, to enable her to better communicate to those in addiction, that recovery is possible. She not only instils hope but also how to change lifestyles.

Sarina highlights in this book the progression of the illness – that is encompassed in 'Addiction'. How people live in denial, secrecy and hide in 'plain sight'. This self-deception in active addiction, before help is sought is of course so damaging to the addict, their families and friends.

She addresses a variety of issues in the book including, enabling, insomnia, triggers for relapse, cravings, processing anger and the major topics of recovery, acceptance, relapse and re-building lives after treatment. She seeks to help those in the grip of addiction, to not only survive and endure, but to recover. Not only does she write from enormous clinical experience, but it is also a lived experience too.

I strongly commend Communication and Connection to you.

Best wishes in your journey, whether you are someone in active addiction seeking help; or the relative or loved one who need help too.

My very best wishes to you.

Dr Simon Kelly Consultant Psychiatrist
MBBS MSc(Psych.) FRCPsych.

Preface

Will you listen to me?

Can we communicate, and can we connect? The title of this book after all is relevant in considering if you can listen, hear, and connect to what I will be talking about. Addiction and recovery is a great passion of mine. I lived in the grips of an out-of-control addiction for approximately 15 years. I knew in this time I was not a 'bad' person but sometimes my behaviour whilst under the influence of drugs or alcohol turned me into someone I was ashamed of being. Not a good thing to feel, it left me depressed and hopeless at times as I tried to figure out how to hide what I was doing. I loved my mother and family but had to escape her knowing eyes on me. She was the first person ever to call my behaviour out for what it was. I developed a habit which is called a geographical in the recovery world, a running away from the present problems, imagining things would be different in another town, country etcetera.

It was not all awful of course, as the behaviour led me to some fantastic places, and I have lived in France, Australia, Jersey, Holland as well as England. Trouble followed me however to those distant lands and the out of control addict me resurfaced in every place I went to. It took time for others to see who I was, and to experience some of my crazy, but always in the end, the me I despised was seen. A series of painful life events led me to my rock bottom and in desperate need of rescue. No white knight for me but rescue never the less came in the form of other addicts who had somehow managed to stop their destructive use and were living 'normal' lives.

Today I am happy to tell you I have been clean and sober for over thirty years. I found the people to help me first in the rooms of Alcoholics Anonymous and Narcotics Anonymous and then in extensive therapy. Remember I was 'crazy'. I met many people along the way to here and now, who have been guides and mentors, wonderful generous souls who asked nothing in return from me except to be clean and sober and to quieten the unrest in my soul.

Along the winding journey of recovery another set of circumstances pushed me into training to be a therapist. I often say it is three things that have saved my life, first of all was AA, then personal therapy and then my training to be a therapist. All these things forced me into looking at and healing the great chasms in my soul, created when things were not as they should have been in childhood. AA, therapy, and training have been instrumental in keeping me clean, sober, and changing. I talk to others daily about how to change, about how to stop destroying self, about how to understand the many things that addiction can teach us. I have also learned how to quiet my unrest, and to nourish my soul.

I have trained in and become accredited as an addiction professional. I continue to study and learn about this perplexing monumental disease. I want the world to change its mind about addiction, to see it as a mental health problem, which needs treating and not punishing. I want perceptions about addiction to change and to this end have written and published other books on the subject. I have discovered that in the healing of self and in order to keep recovery for myself I have to 'give it away'. It is in this amazing process of recovery and sharing it with others I have finally found the me I should have been at the start. The better version of myself. It takes many things however to keep what I have found, as the lure of euphoria is seductively strong. Even after all these years I can still sometimes catch myself thinking that 'perhaps I'm not really an addict', with the unspoken ending being 'so perhaps one or some wouldn't hurt' I know enough about the addict mind and myself today to know that only an addict would think like this. Non addicts don't have this kind if thinking. They don't ponder the question at all.

Today my life is vastly different to the one stumbling from one disaster to another, never listening to anyone's counsel except my own. Today I take pride in the work I can achieve. I am consistent and dependable. People trust me to do what I say I will do. I turn up and am accountable. I also have many wise and wonderful people who I communicate and connect with. In fact I could not do the work I do successfully without those people.

The version of me that existed in the throes of addiction exhibited none of these things. Life today can be difficult, and along with the rest of the world I have had to negotiate the pandemic and its limitations. Having observed the stress and loneliness this imposed. It showed in frightening detail how much we all really need the ability to communicate and connect. This recent world experience clearly demonstrates the need we all have to feel a sense of freedom and possibility to keep our mental health in optimum condition.

As I have continued to refine my sobriety I have discovered that one of my strongest passions is for the ability to translate the freedom I have found into words that will enable others to receive this gift. All this of course began and continues with communication and connection.

Words can heal but can also wound. It is essential therefore we learn how to be truthful and gentle in equal measure. Our communication as healers should be tempered with a desire to do good. We need to set our intentions but not become frustrated when they are ignored or 'thrown away' We cannot force our truth on anyone, we cannot make anyone stop using or destroying themselves with an addiction, all we can really do is show the path forward if an individual wants to walk it.

This way of working with the mental health of addicts is actually the only way I have found to be effective. In my early years learning to be a therapist working with addiction, I was taught that a firm hand and strict discipline was the most effective way. Most treatment centres used to believe that it was beneficial to 'strip people down' in order to 'build them up'. In my experience this method tended to, at best frighten some people away or create excessive self-willed stories that to all intents and purposes served nobody very well. The patient rebelled against the strict discipline or walked away. Who wins in scenarios like this? Only the addiction.

Our skill as teachers, therapists and as people in recovery can really save lives. But once we begin to function as though it is our wisdom and knowledge that is creating the changes, we actually lose our effectiveness. Humility needs to accompany whatever we do with people trying to find recovery.

Whenever I feel or see ego taking over, I remember my own journey to health and sanity. It was a massive gift given to me, yes I needed to 'take it' listen and follow direction but it was nothing clever on my part. I was just able to hear what others said to me. For this ability I am truly grateful. What I 'know' today and what I teach today comes from these humble beginnings. I want to give back; I want also to be able to change perceptions about the disease of addiction. I want to be able to communicate well and to connect with whomever I am talking to.

So will you listen to me? Can we communicate and connect?

Prologue

There are many books written about relapse prevention, clever minds wrestling with this phenomenon of the recovery world. Why do some people 'get' the message of recovery and stay well, and some do not? It is a question that most people who are in recovery from addictive substances or behaviour ponder. It is a question of course that most concerned therapist's contemplate.

I am both, a person in long term recovery from addictive substances and also a therapist collaborating with people in rehab. I ponder this question a lot.

I do wish there were a definitive answer to the question, and that my book goes on to save thousands of lives. It is not exaggeration to talk about saving thousands of lives. As the disease of addiction claims thousands, and as the years go by, the numbers do not lessen but grow. No, there is not a definitive answer, yet I do believe there are answers. These are not simple or just one answer but are contained in the many different and sometimes obscure things a person contemplating a recovery has to do and think about. It is the continued application of these things that creates success.

This book will explore some of those diverse things. The book is entitled Communication and Connection which I propose are two particularly important aspects of recovery from addictive substances and behaviours. Even though it is just the beginning, without them you cannot travel far. So communicate what? And connect with whom? We will look at the things that need to be communicated about, and with whom we should connect with in order to do it. One without the other renders each useless or ineffectual. Most addict can talk quite well, are good orators when it is needed, few know how to listen, or follow directions. Most addicts have many people they can connect with, however some of the people in the practising addicts life end up being just the sort of influence they should not spend too much time with. We are all creatures of habit, we tend to want to be around others who do similar things, like similar things to us. Most addicts keep part of themselves secret even from their spouses, partners, or best friends, especially if they do not share an addiction themselves.

As the disease progresses and the behaviours become more out of control it is not unusual for the addict to choose isolation as their preferred place of 'safety'. It is another reason that the addicts thinking, and actions appear so bizarre at times. In the illness, those who have it, know that some of the time the behaviour is questionable, so isolation becomes a desirable place to live. It is not just physical isolation, but an isolation that affects mind and soul as well as body. Addicts become shape shifters, changing self to fit with whatever is needed. They can be present but distracted, their minds somewhere else. They certainly become adept at lying, using smoke and mirrors to conceal so much. Is it any wonder then, that addicts need to learn how to connect and communicate for change to happen?

We will explore all of these things and discuss addiction which is at the core of everything about this book. Without an understanding of the disease concept, there is very little else that will make much sense about the way addicts need to change and to continue to find ways to remain focused. Recovery does take work and application, some of which people have great difficulty doing unless they understand how serious an illness addiction can be. We will contemplate the brain and the mind and just what might be wrong when addiction is the powerhouse. We will look at soul and spirituality, which are concepts sometimes foreign at the start of recovery but become essential and exciting when the illness is managed, and the muddled brain of the addict begins to experience acceptance and life. I have asked others to write some of their thoughts about the subject to give texture and interest and explore just what an important and diverse subject Communication and Connection is.

Angie Cullen

Family Liaison Support – RMN – Addiction Therapist

I always felt alone as a child, at home I disappeared into books from the age of 4/5 – sitting quietly sucking my thumb in a corner. At school I was initially extremely shy and bullied – 'sit on that wall and don't move' – so I didn't. Other children came up to me and then I could be bright and bubbly and full of questions. The grown-ups were a different matter. Both my parents were alcoholics – Dad a GP with a strong work ethic and huge aspirations – a very clever man but big and scary. Mum very shy but quite strict. We moved 10 times to always bigger and grander houses – 10 schools – there were 3 of us (younger brother and sister) we were not asked how we were, just told to be good soldiers. I could make friends but never keep them. I could do the superficial polite stuff very well but never found out what happened after that.

Last school, a huge Notting Hill Comprehensive where I just got lost – in every way – I had already started smoking cannabis and taking LSD with the friends in my last tiny school. We lived in Chelsea then so at the age of 13/14 I rapidly wanted to be part of the flower power hippy in- crowd, and right there I had found my tribe with whom I started communicating and connecting.

Less and less school for this clever girl who had been near the top of her classes. I started dealing drugs to the rich and famous at the tender age of 16. The famous saying is if you remember the 1960's you weren't there – I can't remember the 60's.

Fast forward to 1981 – Rehab – 'Do you want help?' – Yes - New Tribe.

'How do you feel?' I had no ability to even say that I didn't know. Eventually being scared of being kicked out of this place that I instinctively felt at home in, I asked them to help me – they did. I learnt some of the words to what I was feeling - fear, anger, shame, guilt, disappointment, confusion and hurt.

A rebirth.

I had been chained by what others thought of me, expected of me and what I thought they wanted me to say or do. I was different with everyone, desperately trying to please. Who was I?

I found out in the forty-one years of working a recovery programme and learning how to honestly communicate and connect.

1:

The Disease Concept

Alcoholism, drug addiction, (legal and illegal) and numerous things such as nicotine, caffeine, even sugar are all substances that can be addictive, some more dangerous than others, but all harmful to the human body if taken in quantity. There are also behavioural addictions, such as gambling, gaming, food addictions, (Overeating, Anorexia, and Bulimia), sex addiction, and all manner of things found on the internet such as pornography, social media, plastic surgery and many more behaviours that when out of control become harmful to the human body, mind, and spirit. For all the many different substances and out of control behaviours I shall call them 'addictions' and for ease of understanding the people with addictions are called 'addicts'. Of course looking at each particular thing separately we have alcoholics, drug addicts, gamblers etcetera, but they all have **addictive behaviour**. I use the term to highlight that this illness is much more than the name of the substance or action. It is often stated that calling it a disease is simply an excuse for bad behaviour. I hope to dispel that idea.

So what is addiction? Let us play detective.

It is now well documented that addiction can be classed as a disease; it is:

Primary – there is a genetic component to it that means it is present at birth. It was present from the start. It needs certain things to flourish, things such as (environment/culture/individual biology) but once it is activated it remains in its active state until recognised and managed. It is present sometimes with other illness's which also need treating. Depression, Anxiety, ADHD, Personality Disorder, and many others can be present. This is known as 'Dual Diagnosis'. In Rehab all illnesses need treating, it is not unusual for an addict to have been battling with many other illnesses, and perhaps using the addiction in order to self-medicate. If abstinence and recovery is to be achieved everything the individual has been going through needs to be treated.

Chronic – it has usually been present for a long time and will continue to progress until some of the damaging symptoms are recognised as addiction. It also depicts there is no known cure.

Progressive – It remains as an active dangerous compulsion and will eventually destroy the person who has it if it remains untreated. It becomes worse in its progression. Physically certainly but also mentally. Emotional responses become dysfunctional and there are diminished recognition of problematic behaviour.

Fatal – the progressive nature of this illness means unless it is recognised and managed the person who has it will continue to use until stopped by severe illness or death, with behaviours and thinking continuing to become increasingly compromised. Liver disease, heart disease, cancer, suicide, accidents, and many other tragic consequences might have been prevented if addiction were not present or could have been halted.

Addicts experience loss of control, craving, persistent use despite negative consequences, decision making deficits and loss of insight.

It is one of the most perplexing and bizarre illness's. There are problems with perception, learning, impulse control, compulsivity, and judgement. Despite concerns expressed by others, ability or desire to change is low, and addicts the world over have little awareness of the magnitude of the problem.

Research has shown there is a genetic predisposition to addiction. **A mechanism exists that transmits environmental information from one generation to the next**. Research describes trauma and environmental catastrophise such as war or any kind of destruction or stressors as being transmitted from mother to child in utero. Trauma and addiction go hand in hand and can be seen in one generation, not the next, in one twin not the other, in one family member and not the other. It is varied and complex. It is seen as, but is **not**, a weakness or the individuals 'fault'. It means that with the addictive gene the brain is hardwired to developing addiction once activated. It manifests as craving for the substance or behaviour, loss of control over its use and dependence on it despite adverse consequences. Nobody starts out intending to develop addiction, of course not, but many people get caught in its trap. There is a pleasure principal where the neurotransmitter dopamine communicates the feeling which goes from liking to wanting to needing in the reward centres of the brain. Addictive behaviours and substances provide this pleasure principal without any effort involved, and the brain receives a 'better than expected' reward. Over time dopamine creates less effect on the brain, so the person needs to take more of the substance, this develops tolerance which coupled with compulsion becomes another never-ending disaster, on the brain, the body and life. The hedonic setpoint in individuals with the illness changes and the damage creates a scenario where things once enjoyed diminish, and so the person experiences low moods or depression. Addiction is now known to change both brain structure and function. To break its hold on individuals there are multiple strategies that must be used, psychotherapy, medication, education and of course self-care. Impossible to break the problem if the addict stays isolated.

Dopamine-releasing chemicals

Alcohol/Sedatives/Hypnotics

Opiates/Opioids

Cocaine, Amphetamines

Entactogens (MDMA)

Entheogens/Hallucinogens

Dissociates (PCP. Ketamine)

Cannabinoids

Inhalants

Nicotine, Caffeine, Sugar

Anabolic-Androgenic Steroids

Dopamine-releasing Behaviours

Food (Bulimia, anorexia, Binge Eating)

Sex/Chem sex

Relationships

Tattooing/plastic surgery

Other People (Co-dependency, Control)

Gambling

Performance (Workaholism)

Collection/Accumulation (shopping)

Rage/Violence

Media/Entertainment

Addiction to Codeine

This has become such a problem that it is worth a special mention. The industry is seeing more and more people with out-of-control addiction to codeine who are seeking treatment. When used correctly it is an effective pain suppressant. But as with most other things that people get hooked on, it has a euphoric and anesthetising effect, this, as well as the ability to purchase it over the counter and relative cheapness make it something to be wary of. In America of course the opioid pandemic is well documented, with deaths from and ruined lives talked about. We in the UK are rapidly following suit. Multiple stories exist where people travel from chemist to chemist to be able to purchase enough of the drug and also to hide their identities from the sales people. This resembles stories that alcoholics have told for years. This behaviour is interesting as it shows how determined an addict can be but also perhaps the need to conceal which depicts shame in what they are doing.

Another abundant neurochemical found in the brain is something called Glutamate – this chemical is critical in memory formation; all drugs of abuse and many addicting behaviours affect Glutamate which preserves drug memories and creates drug cues. It also is the neurochemical of motivation, it initiates drug seeking.

McCauley K, MD 2016
Neurobiology of Addiction & Recovery

Symptoms of all illnesses are found in the diagnostic tools (DSM IV) that doctors use to classify illness and disease of which addiction is just one. Other manuals that also describe addiction are freely available. Addiction is known, yet not known, another strange anomaly about this disease is that the illness is still seen as a selfish self-inflicted thing, or a choice. Some people still think it is a 'cop-out' to call it an illness. Perhaps if everyone could understand what it takes to become and stay sober this may change?

Much research continues on this devastating disease, however, to date there has been no way found of curing it or stopping its progress once activated. It is not all doom and gloom however as many with the illness have found a way of keeping the illness dormant and managed. If it is treated in the right way there are solutions. It is recognised as a disease by the World Health Organisation, and by the medical profession. The harmful degrading things that occur in active addiction can be halted, but abstinence alone will not completely halt the damaging thoughts, feelings, and behaviours.

Research has discovered that part of the problem lies in the brain. The incredible piece of kit that we call the brain is flawed in addicts. In a percentage of the population, those amongst us who have the addictive gene, 'switch' on this defect when we take the first drink or drug. The same part of the brain is activated without any substances with behavioural addiction. The 'choice' mechanism is faulty, with the need for the drug or the behaviour that creates dopamine and obsessive use becoming more dominant than it is in others without the gene. This explains why some people can use alcohol or drugs with no seeming ill effect, and others destroy their world in the out-of-control usage. Because not everyone's experience is the same and some people can use with impunity, the door is wide open to stigmatise those with the faulty gene and call them selfish, shameful, or criminal rather than sick. So in this difficult scenario our hapless addicts have to find answers quickly.

Addicts also have certain traits that are in play sometimes long before any addiction has manifested. Studies about addiction have discovered something called sensory augmentation, in other words super sensitivity. It is this sensitivity that sometimes becomes the reason and/or excuse for the drinking or drugging etcetera to start and continue. A mood altering chemical or addictive behaviour can quickly soothe the most sensitive of persons mind or quell the stress of anyone.

It is the success of the addiction for the addict that marks out the difference between addicts or non-addicts. For non-addicts, the same things may be ingested or done with very different outcomes.

Abstinence is the first aspect of a recovery journey that needs to be achieved, sometimes with medical help, but this alone cannot alter habitual patterns of behaviours or obliterate the feeling self, which more often than not have reached despairing places, becoming worse when the solution to all ills (the addiction) is stopped. Abstinence too is the very thing most addicts cannot contemplate. In order to understand this we must understand the relationship addicts have with their drug or behaviour of choice. It is a friend, a need, a comfort when things go wrong, a social lubricant and everything that calms the jittery minds of the people who have this illness. It is the answer and the problem, and at first the addict cannot see the problem, only the answer.

Brain abnormality is a very simple explanation as to what goes wrong in the addict, more information about the brain will be discussed as we continue our detective work, there will also be many references in the resources section of this book.

The brain of course is the power house of human beings, we think, feel and act using our brain. So if the mechanism is faulty, then our thoughts, feelings and actions become faulty. This is where the idea of communication and connection can be understood to be some of the most important aspects of recovery if an addict is to discover solutions to the problems in their lives and to stay well.

An addict will usually only seek help for the condition of addiction when the consequences of using have become out of control and unbearable.

There may have been many signs and symptoms along the way to admitting there is a problem, but the faulty thought mechanism of the practising addict will find a way to justify and minimise until there is nowhere else to run or hide. Many addicts who seek recovery have had catastrophic losses and damage along the way to surrender. Those who do, will survive, those who do not, die lonely ugly deaths with increased disaster being gathered along the way.

Collateral Damage

They say that addicts affect at least six other people in their lives. So with out-of-control behaviour becoming the norm for most addicts, most people in the addicts life can also become adversely affected. In family systems the dynamics can be dangerous and harmful, which was seen very clearly with panoramic view in our recent world-wide pandemic when lockdown forced people into unnatural living arrangements when the usual social interactions stopped, and people were 'forced' into living closely together. It was reported in news articles that the sale of alcohol increased alarmingly as did the incidences of domestic abuse. Now not all addicts of course become abusers of other people, but the act of out of control using itself means that perception and control are compromised. Some drugs might make one more impulsive, more obsessive, and sometimes more aggressive, behaviour in addiction sometimes spiral becoming worse over time. This happens pandemic or not, which leaves the possibility wide open for the faulty decision making of the out-of-control addict to behave in ways that defy logic.

Many addicts end up with a caseload of behaviours they are ashamed about. This of course has to be worked on in a systematic way. No-one can live happy contented lives with a secret stash of unreasonable or shameful behaviour in their history.

Blackouts which are an early feature of the illness for some alcoholics mean that at times a person under the influence can do unbelievable things and have no memory of it. A blackout is an incredibly creepy phenomenon, it is not passing out, or becoming unconscious, yet it is a complete shutdown of the awareness part of the brain, with no physical signs this is happening. So an individual can look normal, perhaps sound normal, and do fairly normal looking things, as well as acting bizarrely at times. They cannot remember however when they 'come to' what exactly they did do or say. Not all behaviour will be normal however and there have been serious crimes committed in blackout and the knowledge of whatever took place never becoming known to the addict, but the consequences because of the actions still have to be played out in real time. The insanity of my own using was to take another substance, usually an amphetamine or cocaine in order to be able drink without blacking out. I never thought about not using at all. This never struck me as crazy behaviour until I viewed it from the side of recovery and sanity. Now I can see how dangerous this was. Yet addicts do this kind of stuff all the time without thinking too much about it. Interestingly if blackouts were seen as one of the first indications of addiction perhaps more people would be alerted to a massive problem brewing. Unfortunately, blackouts are mainly seen as 'just one of things that depict a good night out' accepted as part of the 'good times' addicts think they are having. Blackouts are dangerous, sometimes deadly, and unfortunately ignored as one of the first symptoms of addiction.

Blackouts or not, as the bad behaviours become progressively more frequent it is not unusual for addicts to be severely depressed and incredibly anxious.

Most of the substances themselves are depressants, even with uppers such as cocaine etcetera there are monumental crashes in mood. As the cumulative effect of depressant drugs and awful behaviour increase, it is not unusual for an individual to wonder what is the point of life and to seek a way out. Suicide, sadly is a terrible consequence of some peoples addiction. It is reported that many 'successful' suicides have one substance or another as the driver to the act. Shocking and sad though this is, the statistics imply that this is on the increase, with younger and younger people opting for this permanent solution to whatever their temporary issues are. When in the 'temporary problem' however one never realises it, the despairing feelings just stretch far into the future and the disturbed brain has no way of escaping this if left to its own devises.

Fragile minds and souls often look for the quickest ways to end the problems without realising the echoes of despair and sadness their actions will create in the lives of those left behind for years and perhaps forever. In blackout however the act can be played out with no real awareness. It is debateable on many levels whether the minds of practising addicts can be classed as sane. Playing mind-detectives we will examine some of this in subsequent chapters and come hopefully to new conclusions.

Shocking, harmful, dangerous and one in ten (conservative) of the population have the illness. A pandemic of epic proportions in itself. Yet so much misinformation exists about addiction and so many arguments about how to treat it. The answer to this conundrum of course is to be found in the history of treatment itself and the many attempts of people trying to treat the illness. The fact that the stigma continues is testament to the complex nature of the illness and sadly is the reason many fail or do not access help early on. Remember the addict usually only seeks help when all other avenues are closed. The fact that the solution to the illness has to begin with abstinence is another reason so many people fail to get help and stop. In the faulty thinking of the addict lies the belief that the solution to all their woes is the using itself.

The euphoric prize in addiction is what keeps the addict using and the idea of stopping is something that does not make sense. Most humans seek to feel happy and contented, for the addict, happy and contented is found in the using of an addictive substance or behaviours. The fact that in the progression, the happy and contented stance is lost and the using simply enables the addict to function normally is not something acknowledged. It has to be discovered or pointed out in the recovery process.

Once the using stops being simply a social thing and changes to the thing done when stressed or life gets tricky is the time addicts need to realise that the using has changed into something much more serious. It is no longer a social lubricant, but a panacea for all ills. Strange to think that this one tiny truth if understood could alter what happens next. Unfortunately by the time this change in modus operandi happens, clear thinking or common sense has escaped, and the denial systems are completely in charge of the brain.

There are many modalities of treatment for addiction, my primary discussion will reflect on what is known as the Minnesota method or 12-step way. I use this method in my own life and also know of many recovering people who have decades of 'clean-time' using this method. I never decry anything that works in addiction treatment, what will work for one will not for another. However I can talk about my own experience of recovery, tell examples of countless people who remain well using this method, and hopefully guide others to find solutions for themselves.

The 12-step method or Alcoholics Anonymous, or any of

the Anonymous meetings that exist are often misunderstood. They are described as religious programmes or cults. The language of the programme certainly would give anyone who views it initially or who skims the surface, or who sees it and runs away, the idea that it is religious. What we know about the programme was that it was written 90 years ago, by two men (alcoholics) who were Christians, they were smart cookies these two and so the wording of the programme talks about God or a Power greater than self that has to be found. It is as if they knew that the obstacle for some addicts in accessing the programme would be the 'god word,' so they went to great lengths to talk about whatever the belief system a person has will work as long as it was not just self in the equation. So in the fellowship today you have Buddhists, Christians, Atheists, and all manner of beliefs which all can work, if integrated with the 12-step programme. It is called 'a simple programme for complicated people'. To find out more about any of this, the Alcoholics Big Book is recommended reading. However, do not try to read it alone, you will come across much that is often misunderstood, so the best way to read it is with someone else who already knows something about the programme and will explain it to you.

The incredible thing is that the programme will work for anyone who wants it to. The God word is often spoken about with people who are more knowledgeable trying to explain it is simply a three-letter word that can describe whatever belief/faith/ideas about life that you have, something like, group of drunks or druggies, good orderly direction, or indeed a religious God if that is what you believe in. The salient point of the God discussion is that there needs to be a power greater than self because in the case of addiction the power an individual has, such as self-will and determination is ineffective against the disease. Hence the understanding that the power for a solution lies outside of self. Learning how to communicate and connect with this power is what keeps addicts sober and well. Learning about the brain and how to keep it 'behaving' is another must, and none of this happens if the addict stays isolated. They do not have the answers, they need others to point things out, and run things by.

My intuitive self gets goose bumps when I think about how close I came to missing the amazing knowledge passed down by those two men and the first struggling members of the organisation called Alcoholics Anonymous. If they had not created the programme, or I had walked away from it are moments in time that I call miraculous.

I refuse to argue about wording or whether it is correct to call the organisation a 'fellowship,' or stress about if it is religious. I have made peace with the old-fashioned language Some people in the world will argue about such things and I am not saying sometimes things like that are not important to argue, but in this case what the programme gives in return is worth all the non 'woke' language. I have a miracle that occurred in my life, and no-one can dissuade me from this belief or change the gratitude I and millions of others have about the programme.

AA ---The Lodestar

We can be grateful for every agency or method that tries to solve the problem of alcoholism – whether of medicine, religion, education, or research. We can be open minded towards all such efforts, and we can be sympathetic when the ill-advised ones fail. We can remember that AA itself ran for years on 'trial and error'.

As individuals we can and should work with those that promise success – even a little success.

***

Every one of the pioneers in the total field of alcoholism will generously say that had it not been for the living proof of recovery in AA, they could not have gone on. AA was the lodestar of hope and help that kept them at it.

Grapevine March 1958
The AA Way Of Life Bill W

Anne Barton
Retired Head Teacher and Leadership Consultant

My alcohol addiction was characterised by isolation. I rarely made or took phone calls, and all too often texts and emails were left unanswered. Social arrangements were avoided whenever possible, and I didn't answer the door unless I knew it was a delivery. Without any social contact, there was no need to pay attention to my appearance and I could waste the entire day on meaningless and unproductive activities.

This behaviour all developed after my retirement. During my working life, the discipline of my timetabled life and love for the profession I was in, enabled me to restrict my alcohol use to my free time. I never allowed myself to lose the discipline whilst at school.

Once retired though, I lived in a secret hell of my own making: the all-consuming addiction progressed rapidly and left no room for anything else. I was depressed, ashamed and, although I would vehemently deny it, beaten by alcohol.

When finally I did admit defeat, I took the decision to sign up for 28 days of residential addiction treatment. I accepted it would be tough and I baulked at the prospect of group therapy. Despite my previous professional attributes where running meetings were the norm for me, 'group therapy' was a terrifying prospect. In my opinion, one-to-one therapy would be far more productive. This was self-delusion. In the past I had signed up through my GP for some counselling, not mentioning of course the root cause of my depression, namely addiction. I danced through the sessions, spinning yarns, and entertaining the counsellor. At the end of the sessions I told her I felt so much better and continued to drink.

I learnt that in group therapy there was no-where to hide, we were all clinging onto the life-raft and the stakes were very high. When listening to a fellow patient read aloud some of their work, hearing all the agonising pain, it was impossible not to identify and connect. Being trusted by someone at their most vulnerable, gave me courage and hope. I could be honest no-matter how humiliated and ashamed I was.

Despite this experience, my early days in the fellowship were not so positive. I often thought 'how has it come to this?' I was told to look for the similarities, but I focused on the differences and the resulting alienation was of my own making. In truth, perhaps I had not yet fully accepted my illness. I was often silent or, when I did speak, briefly said what I thought others wanted to hear.

It took several months and on-going therapy before I could trust myself and the groups. I learned that being open in front of others was liberating and it was this that formed strong connections.

I wouldn't be sober today were it not for the peers I continue to communicate and connect with. Having grown up as the child of an alcoholic, I learned the communication rules needed for survival: 'Don't trust, don't talk, don't feel' Today I practice the exact opposite and the communication skills needed for a happy sober life.

2:
Communication and Connection
(Part One)

Communication: transmission, conveyance, divulgence, disclosure, dissemination…

Connection: link, relationship, relation, interconnection, association, bond, tie…

Such 'clunky' words, with a wealth of meaning, I am using them to portray what is one of the most essential aspects of success in anyone's recovery. Every story of recovery, of course has within its creation the story of a relentless, progressive, chronic illness that is known as the disease of addiction.

To communicate effectively we have to have some kind of rapport. Without this anything we communicate can be misunderstood. Addicts tend to look as though they are paying attention, but in actual fact they may be somewhere else entirely. A frustrated spouse who is attempting to illicit understanding that this time the behaviour is too much, may plead and beg the addict to stop destroying the relationship. This will be viewed as nagging, or over-reaction, making connection impossible. No meeting of minds in this conversation. The mental gymnastics of some who are attempting to construct an acceptable narrative is what stops them from really hearing. Part of that is they do not want to hear but part of it is also their brains are unable to really understand due to the many chemical dances that are taking place. If they have already used a substance the dance is powered by the drug, dopamine and serotonin, the feel-good chemicals are released and spikes of many other things also take place, rendering our addict in a mind altered state. They can look the same as ever, but they are mentally elsewhere. With their brains resembling pin ball machines with synapsis firing in all directions. The behaviours of practicing addicts often do not look sane to them, let alone to spouses, employers and concerned friends. We know today of course they are not exactly sane; the addiction is in control and dictates what happens next. Addicts need to understand that one cannot NOT communicate, there is always some message being received by the people they are in contact with. Sadly, the unspoken message many family members receive is that they are not important, and certainly not as important as the next fix or drink. It is often not what the addict intends to be communicated, but as every gesture, silence or word has multiple meanings, it is easy for everyone to feel and be mis-understood. The addict is looking for the 'feel good' state and often cannot understand what all the fuss is when they start using again. Remember, non-addicts do not experience addiction the same way. It is only in the 'come down' if the behaviour is remembered in a sober state that any kind of remorse will be felt. If the addiction is of long duration, the only feeling left will be to feel normal as soon as possible. The body and mind have taken a huge assault again when a binge is playing out, so the getting back to normal may take days, lots of pain medication and sleep. The aftermath for everyone can resemble a battlefield of emotions. None of them good. This is the life of practicing addicts, doing it again and again. Is this sanity?

ADDICTION - A Reliance on a substance and /or behaviour in order to change the way one feels

It is not simply the over-indulgence of certain substances, some legal, some not, or out of control behaviours around gambling or relationships etcetera, it is much more than that. Feelings, attitudes, beliefs, value systems, self-esteem – EVERYTHING becomes involved when describing the disease of addiction, as these are the very things that become corrupted, broken, or lost as the disease progresses.

The disease of addiction by its very nature thrives in secrecy and isolation. The word denial is often used in describing why the addict cannot stop or see what the rest of the world can easily detect. There has to be secrecy, there has to be isolation, there has to be denial, in order to continue to use in the way the addict wants to. 'If you see me doing this, If I realise what it is doing to others, If I see the truth, I will not be able to continue. I am enthralled by a substance which is mind altering,' such as alcohol, cocaine, heroin, amphetamine, ketamine, methamphetamine, crack, LSD, nicotine, sugar, caffeine, steroids, prescription and over the counter pills and potions. You know this list stretches on for a long, long time, and new substances crop up constantly Will the world ever stop manufacturing substances that alter the mind, or will some individuals ever want to stop using such things?

Probably not!

Addicts also do not want to be told that what they are doing is crazy or wrong, and they of course never talk about the way they feel about using substances or engaging in something that makes them feel invincible.

Equally some can be addicted to behaviours which alter brain chemistry in similar ways to mind altering substances, things such as gambling, gaming, sex, cosmetic surgery, tattooing, social media, pornography, exercise, spending/shopping or eating disorders, from bulimia to anorexia and overeating the same part of the brain becomes activated using these behaviours and addiction develops in the pursuit of what the actions feel like. As things such as sex and relationships and some of the other mentioned acts are natural and engaged in as a normal part of life, it is important to remember that addiction is present when the behaviour becomes out of control and unmanageable. Again the list of things we can be addicted to goes on and on. Will some individuals ever want to not do these things?

Probably not!

Also as some of these things are done by most people, the problematic usage only becomes visible when life becomes unmanageable, or something catastrophic happens to stop the addict in his/her tracks. Until then it is assumed 'that everyone does it, how can it be bad for us?' Remember not everyone has the addictive gene and faulty brain chemistry, not everyone's behaviour and use of the substances or behaviours becomes out of control,

So the question should be, 'what can be done about addiction, is it possible to track and trace, is it possible to stop its relentless progression in some people's lives?' Imagining a scenario where an App is created that will tell the user that your brain is not functioning well and your solution to your stresses make it worse, it seems farfetched and sci fi like, however science and technology have come a long way already, so that in the future such things could be invented. At one time brain imagery was a distant dream, nowadays it is common place to be able to scan the brain and see how it is functioning. Sadly for now Apps to discern poor brain functioning do not exist. We have to rely on other means to try to get well and stay well. We have to rely on others to tell us what is wrong.

It is well documented these days that what is wrong with addicts can be viewed as abnormalities in the brain. The 'choice' mechanism in the addicts brain gets hi-jacked by addiction rendering the addict unable to choose not to use, despite at times terrible consequences. This abnormality is not visible without a brain scan, therefore not universally known, and often the addict does not realise they have this abnormality until the addiction is well advanced. By which time of course, the problems and trouble which accompany addiction will be easily detected. But the desire to conceal will be sky high.

What sort of problems or troubles?

1. Trouble such as problems in **relationships,** when the people around the addict can no longer stand the unmanageable nature of their lives. There may be the already documented domestic violence, or simply screaming matches that make home life unbearable. There may be debt, or affairs, or families at war. There may be children who witness things they should never see or hear. Separations, divorces, unhappiness, and desperation, just some of the things that out-of-control addiction can produce.

2. There may be **health problems**, the well- known dangers to the liver are not the only things that go wrong of course. Just about every part of the human body can be adversely affected by the use of alcohol and drugs. Most of the harm done though is unseen and again undetected until late in the onset of the

addiction. Our bodies do not always deal with the relentless abuse poured on it. When we are eighteen perhaps we can cope with the late nights and various substances or behaviours we submit it to. But as these substances can be described as poisonous and the behaviour as destructive, is it any wonder our bodies sometimes object and fail us?

3. Clashes with the **law** are often part of what goes amiss in the lives of addicts. Some of the substances used of course are illegal and obtaining them breaks the law, driving whilst under the influence is a common act. Some people are reduced to stealing or committing crime to fund their addiction. Then the violence and mayhem that out of control using seems to promote go hand in hand with advanced addiction. If alcohol were illegal as the world health organisation believes it should be, there would be many more individuals breaking the law. Yet interestingly this drug is the most easily obtained and can be found everywhere and used for everything, from births to marriages to funerals etcetera. This is despite more deaths from alcoholism that are recorded than from cocaine or heroin. It is my hope that in years to come alcohol will be treated in the same way as nicotine has, they are both killers, but clemency is given to alcohol. The reason alcoholism is treated differently to other drugs is to be found in history and politics. There are many fine books that have been written about the subject which I shall reference later.

4. **Education and work** are often interrupted by some of the out-of-control behaviour. Debt and poor economic management can be a fact in the lives of addicts. Work is usually the last thing to be lost in a

catalogue of losses when it comes to addiction. It is as though the addict knows to hang on for dear life to the thing that funds the only true love of the addicts life. Education/school/college can be interrupted, grades lost opportunities smashed with no-one really knowing why.

5. **Emotional and Mental Health** are often progressively damaged as the illness progresses. There may of course be underlying problems which the addiction are masking, or the addict is using to explain their behaviour. This area is complex but undoubtably the emotional and mental health in out-of-control addiction is something to take notice of. Some of these problems with the mind and emotions can be changed, stopped and recovery found, however with all the physical and mental damage there is a tipping point.

When will it be too late?

It is fact that just about every aspect of life can be affected by addiction and often is, as it progresses in the addicts life. It is usually a crisis in one of these areas that propels the addicted person to stop, look at what is happening because of the addiction and if they are lucky, do something about it. To call it a love affair is not too false a description, it certainly looks like this to anyone who witnesses what is happening in the life of an addict. It never makes sense, looks entirely mad, and can legitimately be called insanity. Not for the 'nutty' things done, but for the 'thinking' that does the same 'nutty' things repeatedly and again, never seeming to learn from the catastrophic carnage the behaviour creates. The addict never seems to learn from the last disaster. The brain and body demands the feelgood stuff and the merry-go-round is entered into.

Spouses, employers, parents, even police and the courts may have issued warning after warning about abhorrent behaviour. The denial that addicts get lost in is so strong that unless a moment of clear sight is reached nothing, but nothing seems to break the spell of addiction. Perhaps it is this fact that makes the term 'illness' or 'disease' so hard to accept. In most other disease's there is usually no issue in wanting and having treatment. Once it is recognised then seeking help and treatment is a fact of life. But with addiction the historical attempts to deal with it or treat it (lobotomy and straightjackets or prisons) become why there is so much misunderstanding around how to deal with it. Information about what goes on in the brain is relatively new information, a lot of things now known have not been known for very long in terms of medicine. Also the denial systems of the practicing addict make it hard to reach them.

Is it not time to change this narrative?

Libby Garnham
Founder/Chairman of ANA Treatment Centres

In communicating with others, we tend to concentrate mainly on what we want to say or get across. In doing this often forgetting that effective communication is more about listening. Listening not only to the words being spoken but to the emotional message being conveyed. Text books tell us communication works when both the sender and the receiver assign similar meanings to the message. Unfortunately, this is rare in a group or room full of individuals who will hear and internalise the message differently. Within groups many barriers come into play, to name a few, culture, language, the use of jargon and acronyms, prejudice's, and the inability to see or read general body language. The list is endless making it quite remarkable that we ever connect. Language can be distorted leading to confusion and misunderstanding. This can also be the case in a one-to-one meeting where the sender and receiver have their own agenda, both set on getting their message across and unable to listen to the other.

Communication, however, is the bedrock of our lives, it is how we get things done, how we explain ourselves and how we express emotion. It is imperative in every walk of life from running a household to acting as an advocate or just being friends. It helps to have some self-knowledge and understand the impact we have on other people. Being thoughtful before speaking, adjusting language, and delivering it to fit with the situation and to whom we are communicating with.

There are many forms of communication other than the spoken word. This can be useful when there is trauma, where there may not be words available to express pain or to speak the unspeakable. Apart from EMDR (Eye Movement Desensitisation and Reprocessing) or EFT (Emotional Freedom Technique), music and art can be incredibly effective in bringing people together and encouraging expression of feelings. The power of music can transform lives, improve the immune system, increase dopamine levels, and reduce stress. Art Therapy encourages the exploration of feelings and helps individuals find meaning and make connections. Both forms of communication can provide healing, that facilitates physical, emotional, cognitive, and social change.

All forms of good communication help bring people together, broaden our knowledge of life, ourselves, and others. However thoughtless and unkind words can destroy confidence, belittle people, bringing misery and hurt. There may be many pitfalls but when used well it gives us the ability to engage, to learn, make friendships and broaden our lives beyond measure.

3:

Communication and Connection

(Part Two)

So what does communication and connection have to do with addiction?

In the progression of the illness of course there is extraordinarily little of either. The addict has to retreat into worlds that house like for like. Has to frequent the places where he/she will not be detected or thought of as 'wrong'. The addict has to find how to hide in plain sight. To do the things they want to do they need to retreat. Sometimes they will become loners in lonely lands, sometimes they will be part of what looks like normality, but always on the outskirts. Mentally distracted or mentally absent. Minds preoccupied with the next fix, or the next lie. Working out how to cover up the deception. What sounds like a good excuse or plan, how not to get found out, or if found out how to cover it up, takes a lot of work. As the disease progresses addicts often become increasingly isolated mentally. What starts out in most addicts lives as a social lubricant actually becomes the thing that separates and destroys all normal socially acceptable life.

The addict then has to hide and isolate if only to protect their 'friend, their love the panacea of all ills' from being taken from them. Most addicts will have encountered those who do not like them using and want them to stop.

They will encounter obstacles at every turn. The only way to protect the addiction is to deny, to lie, to hide and to isolate. It becomes the ingrained behaviour of many addicts. Most do not realise it however, as they can live half-lives, they can hold down good jobs, get married do 'almost' normal things. But always in the background the addiction will be waiting. As the disease of addiction does not have a 'sell by date' the progression can be quick or slow depending on circumstances.

The thinking of the addict becomes twisted and bizarre. You need no imagination to see and understand twisted wires. Because the park bench or the dirty mac and hidden bottles or the junkie in the alleyway are not the image we think of ourselves exhibiting we sincerely believe we cannot be addicts. This stereotype kills more people than anything else. No-one chooses a park bench, sometimes this an enforced living arrangement if the job, the money, and the people who love us have long gone. But for many, those people stick around, or our money protects us and saves us from destitution. Seriously though it is a matter of luck. If it has not happened to you, this is called one of your yet's. Incubate the illness long enough and it may still be a reality.

In order to break out of the denial system that the addict lives in, they have to understand as they reach for help with their addictions, that most cannot and never will be able to find recovery alone. Therefore the first time they reach out for help is the first time they will need to communicate honestly about what has been going on. However this will be useless unless a connection to another person who understands the illness is made. It is at this crucial start of any recovery that communication and connection has to be established. Some can do it some cannot. The disease affects the brain in ways that are hard to understand. The thinking of the addict has been twisted beyond all semblance of normality. It is not seen or understood by the addict themselves so what chance has the public at large, or of the desperate spouse or the angry employer?

No chance at all.

EXAMPLES

1. **On an important business trip to a foreign country. Taken or sent by the boss for the skills and business acumen that normally are in plentiful supply. The 'free' drinks on the flight over followed by 'the quiet night in to prepare' which develops into a bender so ferocious the addict ends up in intensive care needing to be flown home at great expense by the company. It is only the relationship with the boss that saves the job in this instance.**

There is always a next time, and always worse examples of out if control behaviour. Perhaps this was the straw that broke the camel's back as your behaviour and attitudes are recognised for what they really are, and you are sacked. You have become a liability and an embarrassment.

2. **Exams tomorrow are preceded by amphetamines to keep awake and alert, which culminate in the shakes so badly you cannot hold your pen, let alone think straight. You take some weed to straighten out.**

   You fail your exams and need to retake the year. Or just drop out as mental health declines. Everyone's patience wears thin.

3. **A planned fabulous night out with your loved one, starts in the getting ready stage with copious amounts of the preferred drug and continues during the meal, where you are rude to the waiters, and make a fool of yourself over nothing, the ensuing argument on the way home ruins not only the night out but the next weeks or months.**

   Apologies become futile. It re-occurs repeatedly, whilst the promises ensue. Partners feel as if they take second place. The promises are never kept, and the lies become prolific. Until eventually going out together becomes a distant dream.

4. **Weddings, parties, celebrations, you choose to be the designated driver in order to ensure you do not drink. Drinking and driving after all are the worst of the worst. You have 'just one 'with the meal, or to get things going, which ends up with you risking your life and everyone else's as you fail to stop at just one drink.**

   If you are not caught and/or stopped you will go on taking these risks. You will repeat the behaviour despite promising you will not drink and drive. So many people break the law this way by driving after the night before. If they had been breathalysed they would still most definitely be over the limit, and mentally impaired.

5. **You love and respect your partner, but the office party turns into a drunken affair with you breaking your marriage vows over someone whose name you barely know.**

   The ensuing guilt erodes what is a great relationship

both at home with your despairing partner, and at work, with colleagues who you are sure know your dirty little secret. Who do you talk to about this?

6. **One more Grinder session turns into a dangerous 'party' that could threaten life certainly but reputation definitely as everything gets out of hand.**

   The soul sickness after the fact is huge. You take days to recover and contemplate ending your life, things are definitely spiralling out of control.

7. **Just one more bet or roll of the dice wins you the equivalent of an expensive car, your addiction however does not allow you to stop at win, and the next thing you know you have blown next month's mortgage payments.**

   The hardship you and your family experience do not make sense, when only a few minutes ago you were 'rich'.

The confusion in your children's eyes as they witness things children should not see, (or worse) The arguments and lies, the denial and deception take their toll on everyone involved. The progressive nature of the illness plus the development of tolerance for whatever addiction is being pursued renders the addict helpless and powerless to first of all recognise what the problem is and secondly to stop the progression. Everyone in an addicts life is affected, the damage gets worse and worse over time.

The problem is:

1. **I should have eaten before I took those drinks on the plane.**

2. **I should never have stayed up so late cramming before my exams.**
3. **I should have ignored those rude waiters, and my partner looking for a fight.**
4. **I have to delete Grinder and not go back to it.**
5. **I should not have offered to drive, why am always the designated driver?**
6. **I should not have bothered with the office party; predators are always waiting to pounce.**
7. **If only I had stopped when I was winning.**

The deception to self is the most profound, but once it starts it is impossible to stop. You will notice no doubt that the reason for the trouble is always something other than the real culprit. The problem is always something else, someone else. The problem can never be the substance or behaviour. After every shameful experience of course, the using becomes the thing to soothe the fevered shamed self. The drink, the pill or potion, or spending, or whatever the addiction is, becomes the thing to turn to when life becomes problematic, ensuring that the messes get messier, the shame becomes more shameful and the destruction more destructive.

These few examples are a sanitised version of some of the devastation that addiction can bring to an addicts life. What needs to be understood is that although the behaviour looks pretty insane at times especially when it is endlessly repeated. It is not the behaviour that professionals deem insane, but the 'thinking' behind the behaviour. If this can be understood then it is not too difficult a leap for the addict to understand. Some exceptionally brave people have documented and talked about their out-of-control behaviour when under the influence, every one of them could not find a way out of chaos alone.

'If my thinking is like this then perhaps I am not the best person to depend on for an answer to a severe problem such as addiction'

IF ONLY!!

If our struggling addicts could/would think this than half the battle about what to do next and getting out of the dangerous game would not take so long or be so difficult. However the addict and most of the rest of society cannot see this simple truth. Yes the behaviour is seen, and we are aghast, but that the addict has 'thinking' problems is not often considered. That the whole problem of addiction is because of this unseen 'thinking' problem.

This time it will be different,

This time I will only have one line.

This time I will control it

This time I will stop at bet no. 3

This time I will leave at ten o' clock

This time…

The problem with addiction however, and it is never understood in its active stage, is that any involvement with any kind triggers will set off the phenomenon of craving in the addict and at that stage it is almost impossible to limit usage. Addicts cannot find their way out of this tangled mess of trouble and crazy thinking without help. It continues to be trouble incurred outside of self, and if I can fix that all will be well. The help that is needed also needs to be coming from a specific source.

What has been tried in the past?

Many trips to doctors to 'fix' depressions or anxieties or poor sleep or any number of things that go hand and hand with addiction will be pointless if the addiction is not focused on. It rarely is because addicts lie about the root cause, and our overworked GP's do not have time to play detective. The addiction is then overlooked. Our partners and friends also are the wrong people to 'help,' when for years they have lied for us, cleaned up the mess, or even joined in the 'merry-making' in the hope of bringing the relationship closer together. Let us check out our symptoms on Dr Google, let us go to agencies that do harm reduction, teach me to use sensibly. It would only be alcohol that this can be done with of course, as cocaine is illegal as are many other things, and no-one in the right mind would teach you to gamble 'sensibly' if you have a problem. Or use cocaine like a lady. It even sounds crazy yet is thought all the time with the drug called alcohol, it is a potent dangerous drug, which, say the World Health Organisation, ' if discovered today would be a class A drug, dangerous and illegal!' Non-specialist therapies tend to focus and fix other problems like relationship issues and other life issues as these are the triggers, they have to be worked on of course but if the addiction is not dealt with and focused on everything gets sabotaged.

The help one needs has to be from people who understand addiction. AA rooms and specialised addiction therapists and rehab all know about addiction and will steer addicts in the right way. If loved ones or concerned others could have helped I am sure they would have long before now. Anyone in the addicts vicinity has to learn that they are as powerless over their addict as the addict is over the substance or addictive behaviour.

POWERLESSNESS

What does this word imply?

I have no control, something controls me. Anything I try is ineffective.

Are YOU powerless over anything or anyone? Of course we can all say yes to this question, but to actually own up to powerlessness over inanimate things well perhaps we would baulk at this. Powerless over alcohol - really?

We are taught from an early age that autonomy is the desired stance, it shows strength of character. So to admit to 'powerlessness' seems to be a foreign concept. Especially powerlessness over something like alcohol. It is only when an addiction history is written out and contemplated can one see what has actually been visible to everyone else. Powerlessness is the explanation, because if we were not powerless what does that make us? Most of us are not evil or bad. Our behaviours can sometimes look that way. But the drug we easily consume wipes out reason and consideration and we often act in inexplicable ways. Doing this repeatedly and to not expect the same kind of outcomes is what makes us seem insane, and certainly our thinking process could be seen as such.

Once powerlessness can be accepted as the reason our lives become unmanageable well than the next step is to stop taking or doing the thing that creates the powerlessness. As we already examined, seeing what truly is the problem is difficult in a litany of justifications.

None of this comes easily to anyone, the behaviours have become habitual, the thinking done in isolation cannot change, we slip into regular grooves of thinking that cannot change if we stay isolated.

David Musgrave
Managing Director

Before doing something about my addiction, I was completely lost in the world, stuck in a desperate nightmare that I could not find a way out of. My 'escapades' whilst under the influence were becoming more and more dangerous and desperate. I had a moment of clarity whilst in the last nightmare when I knew I had to do something about my addiction or die.

My life was saved in some completely unexpected ways, and by some completely unexpected people.

I was met in the clinic I went to by non -judgemental people who I was able to open up to and tell my story, in all of its technicolour ugliness. These were psychiatrists, doctors and therapists who specialised in addiction. I met other people too who had the same illness as me, with equally shameful stories

I was shocked to learn what was wrong with me and surprised to learn what I needed to do to get well.

I am now two years clean from all mood-altering chemicals. I have begun to make amends to the people in my life that I had harmed. My business and private life are thriving. I am beginning to live a life that had always been closed to me. I grew up furious with the world and by taking my anger out on the world I found myself destroying myself. From a living hell of 20 years to a quiet and spiritual life today, all made possible by stopping the using, addressing my childhood anger, and talking to people who knew me better than I knew myself.

I continue to communicate and connect with specific people. My life still can be problematic but with help all my 'problems' can be dealt with. I am grateful for the gift I have been given so continue to work the programme with the belief that I never have to be that mad stumbling practicing addict again.

4:

Breaking the Denial Trap

Denial – Sincerely believing our own lies

At the end of the progression loop is a place which exists for every addict. The place where self-deception has to end, and the truth has to be seen. Some of course reach it and deny it immediately, but for the lucky ones, me included we hit something which is called our rock bottom. No longer the park bench or junkie with a needle in the arm, the view of popular culture, but a place inside the heart of most addicts, who are perplexed and ashamed about what they see their lives have become. A moment of truth is glimpsed and in some people it is acted on. What do we do in such moments? If we do nothing then eventually the truth fades, and the addiction looks attractive again. If truth is to make the difference and set us free we have to turn to others for help.

Sometimes those we turn to will have the right kind of help for us. In my case I had 'escaped' my mother's view of my drinking, (she never knew about the other drugs) by going to Australia, found most definitely a land of freedom and excitement, where my behaviour mixed in with the Aussie culture seemed to coalesce, which culminated in my addiction progressing fast and becoming out of control. The moment of truth for me led me to ask for help from the organisation known as Alcoholics Anonymous. For some reason I had always known about AA, did not think I needed it of course, but when the chips were down and there was no-one else to turn to this is where I went for help. I was as suspicious of all the religious stuff as anyone else, but the people in the meetings told me not to worry about it and to just stop drinking, come back to as many meetings as possible and wait and see what happens. My first question was how do I not drink? The answer was simple and blunt, 'no-one tips it down your throat' Blunt as only the Australians can be, it simply made sense, and more than sense it awoke something in me that had been dormant, yes of course I can decide not to take the first drink. I had never in all my attempts at trying to control the blackouts ever thought about not drinking. (Another example of flawed thinking?) In fact the only controls I ever tried were to take another mind-altering substance in order to stop the blackouts. All this did of course was make a sick girl sicker and the disease of addiction to be super charged in terms of progression. This sounds ridiculous to me now but was the first light bulb moment amongst many that AA offered me. Now some addicts in the illness could not respond like this as some people cannot for the life of them stop using. But the progression in myself had not yet reached this desperate stage so I was able to stop, I just needed to be convinced it was a good idea, I was also, what is known as a binge drinker/user, so periods of clean time were usual for me. I could never keep it up, however. So asking for help from this organisation was my first serious attempt at stopping and staying stopped. Heavy users or daily drinkers may have a harder time at stopping, and sometimes need medical help to do so.

The first task of arresting this disease is to stop using. We soon learn that this means all the different substances not just the one we used the most often. It is easy to suppose that if I had never tried ecstasy for instance or liked cannabis that it would be ok to use them, as they were not the problem, alcohol and speed were my go to's. However many other people's experiences of doing this had always culminated in relapsing back to their primary. I did not need my own 'proof' I could see it in their desperation and unhappiness that the way back to out of control had to be curbed. I reached these early milestones in a recovery not through my own cleverness or understanding but through other people who knew the way forward out of addiction and into life as life should be. The thing I did right was to listen and to follow suggestions. I do not know why I believed what was being spoken about, but for me it worked, and I shall be eternally grateful that I was able to 'hear'.

At this stage of course we have no understanding about the brain and defective thinking. But most people who reach the doors of AA or NA, or ask for help from a rehab or therapist, understand that something has gone terribly wrong in life. It should never have got to this. The shame and hopelessness all combine to make a depressing awful place to live, the only light is others who understand this place and assure us it will not stay this way if we do certain things. Stay stopped and stay in communication with the people who helped us get clean first of all. We stop listening to our own mixed-up thinking and start listening to others.

There are so many things that need to change in our thinking, but this is where it begins. In a simple admission that we do not have the answers, these new people we meet seem to have some of the answers we want. Many who begin a recovery journey this way are depressed, unhappy, and suspicious. Luckily, our personal rock bottoms and disasters are the things that keep us coming back.

In my life I had reached a point of despising the woman I saw myself becoming in my sober moments. I craved a change; I was desperate to change. I understand now that this state is one of the most powerful states I could have reached and is what kept me in those early days coming back to the programme to learn more. It is a challenging thing to comprehend when one first goes to a meeting, rehab, or therapist, how the hell does listening to others talk about their problems help? Yes an AA meeting does seem weird at first, rehab and therapists less so, yet therapy is still not as accepted as it could be. In all however, the addict will be told to listen and keep coming back. The understanding one needs cannot be gathered quickly. Patience and tolerance are traits one needs

Some cannot achieve any length of sobriety through meetings alone at the start of recovery, so will need to either accept the help from a therapist or rehab, which will give an individual a bit more intensive personal treatment. You know whatever works for whomever is the right way. If they stop a killer in its tracks let us celebrate!

The price of change at this stage is abstinence – this is hard but doable, once addicts understand that it is the first drink or drug that does the damage they will be able to delay that first drink or drug by talking to others and doing any number of things to break the craving for euphoria. They are told to stop mixing with risky people – everyone seems risky at first as these are the people they used with, but gradually and with time they will realise not everyone used the way they did. Not everyone used addictively, some could take it or leave it and what is more will support them in not taking it. Those who cannot stop using will drift away once they realise the addict is serious about not using.

This is a hard truth sometimes, but the culling process happens of its own volition one does not really have to act. Using friends are simply that, people once used with. People with staying power are usually those who truly care for or love us.

Without abstinence there will be no progression in recovery. Sabotage will occur at every level of this journey. The individual will have to stay in dishonesty and denial, nothing said by others will make much sense and the way forward will be totally blocked. Alcohol, drugs, and addictive behaviour will fog the brain and there is nowhere to go with it. Abstinence is a key to a massive change in thinking behaviour but also lifestyle.

This, however, is never easy, other keys are needed and in changing things addicts have to become comfortable with the uncomfortable. Life itself feels awkward, they feel awkward. Things done many times in the past will seem different. There is a cognitive dissonance with things and life. They are not in harmony with the world or their relationships. What has always worked in the past has to change. Mostly of course life improves, but in the improving there are many twists and turns that the addict has no clue how to navigate at first. It is like a foreign land which requires much help from others who have maps and ways out of the maze. The 12 steps are one of the maps that can help. Therapy is another map. There are other maps and ways to help in this journey, but the crucial point is that the individual cannot do it alone. They need to learn to rely on and ask for directions. Sometimes this too is problematic for some individuals, it is though the very thing that will help is a step too far in the recovery journey. Asking for help takes humility, and some addicts egos are so dominant that humility is also a foreign word and place.

In this change of lifestyle, sometimes our lovers and partners decide they do not wish to walk the new paths with us. Or the damage done in the active stage of the story of addiction was so severe and damaging, sticking around for the next episode of a sitcom that appeared to be on 'repeat' is a task too difficult. Letting these people go is hard but holding onto to something that cannot work is harder. If love is truly in the relationship it can survive, but as everyone has to be part of any change it can only happen with much communication and help. The damage done in active addiction is epic and many relationships falter at the early stage of recovery.

Partners, friends and loved ones need to part of the change. It is sometimes misunderstood with words such as 'it is your problem, not mine, you have to work a recovery programme not me'. Easy to understand this thinking, but it too is flawed. Family, friends and loved ones have often had to adapt their behaviour and things they say in order to survive the addicts behaviour. In the support groups for family and friends this is called 'enabling' where the antics and behaviours of the addict are hidden or lied about, all to protect the family and reputation of the addict. Addicts lives are often secretive and very messy and therefore it makes sense that the whole dynamic in the family becomes something not quite right. Some relationships have fared worse than others and will not survive the huge changes that need to happen, if they are to survive then it can only be done with help and communication. There are organisations such as Families Anonymous and Al-anon which function as guides and help for the partners and friends of addicts Many relationships heal through having a mediator help with communication problems. Relate or couples counselling are good choices to help reach better understanding and clear communication. Again this continues the idea that solutions to damaged relationships cannot be found alone. Help is needed and what is more, the exciting thing is, the help that is needed is available and tried and tested.

Children – Part 1

Another lie that has to be dispelled is that the well-defined secrecy in addicts homes protect the children. Not so, sadly young children will either feel frightened when the parent acts badly and they will try to 'disappear,' staying silent so as not to attract attention. Or they grow into resentful angry teens who rebel at the first opportunity. Or both these things! Children are good observers; they witness many things, but they are poor interpreters. They often blame themselves for the bad behaviour in the home. They will feel unheard and unimportant. They will pick up easily the need for secrecy, so nobody gets to hear the fear or confusion the child is dealing with when 'daddy shouts at mummy' or 'mummy falls asleep and burns the dinner'. There are much worse scenarios that happen in out-of-control homes of course, but I'm sure you get the picture. Life is no picture book for these children, and they grow up into people with low self-esteem and a rage that may very well turn into their own more serious mental health issue. If they have the addictive gene of course this may be where they seek solace. They do what they have witnessed at home with their friends, or they resort to self-harming or stealing or shoplifting, or the rebels amongst them will be disruptive, aggressive, or worse.

This last chapter may seem as though life is way too difficult to even contemplate recovery, and in some ways it is at the start, but the compensations of recovery make it eventually a hugely worthwhile venture. In recovery all the previous discussions about what happens in homes, to children, to relationships must be attended to. A newly recovering person will have no clue as to how this can be achieved. Therapy of course is a start, and in recovery rooms up and down the country other people will discuss how they have healed the massive rift in their homes. All of this repair work takes time and patience. It is impossible to turn around the damage caused quickly, and everyone needs help to achieve it.

Lloyd Haylor-Smith
Trainee Therapist

As a recovering addict I have come to understand how vitally important it is to regularly communicate with those who know how it feels to be misunderstood, and by that I mean fellow recovering people. In my active addiction, my love affair with my drugs of choice prevented me from being honest about everything. My only true connection was with myself, but I had no idea who I was without substances. Decades of using had created a personal prison, four feet of cast iron walls in the form of selfishness and bad behaviour.

Today I work a daily recovery programme and those walls have gone. I no longer have to lie to hide my behaviours, which gives me the freedom to communicate with others. Not only other addicts, but also those people dear to me. I love those people and they are now able to love me back.

Early on in my recovery I struggled to connect with others. As I worked the programme I learned that I not yet connected with myself. I was so full of guilt and shame that I hated myself for everything I had been doing. I knew deep down I was capable of loving others, but I did not feel deserving of it. The self-loathing I felt blocked any loving connection, not only with others but also with myself. Whilst in treatment and later on with my sponsor I began the task of finding a power greater than myself. This process took much communication with those in recovery whom I had connected with. This developed into a firm belief that I had found a protective concept that to this day continues to offer protection, forgiveness, and love. This connection requires daily communication. Some call this prayer, but for me, it is not about kneeling and clasping my hands and looking to the sky. It is a 'ritual' I practice as I get ready for the day. I think of everything I am grateful and thankful for and ask for the strength and patience needed for any new or existing challenges. Staying connected this way ensures I remain connected to myself and my feelings. This in turn allows me to communicate with my loved ones, friends, colleagues, and other recovery people and also anyone that I encounter that day. I am reminded that my recovery only exists one day at a time. The day I neglect to connect and communicate is the day my prison rebuilds itself.

5:

Mind and Body

So everything up to this point has been about the preliminary stages of recovery. Recognizing there is trouble in the way life is being led, an acknowledgement that something needs to change. An understanding that try as we might the changes necessary cannot be reached alone.

Addicts have to reach out to others for support and help.

This might be to one of the Anonymous meetings we heard about, to a GP or a rehab or therapist, or someone who knows a bit about what needs to happen to stop using. Whatever the source of help is, the addict needs to ask for the help and do what is suggested.

The first task is to achieve abstinence – if this is not done than nothing else will work. Often addicts will believe the problem is depression or anxiety and try to treat this, without including the whole story. A GP who has not been told the whole story may suspect drinking or addiction is at the heart of the problems but unless the person is willing to be honest, the people trying to help cannot offer the best support. Sometimes a GP will not have the knowledge in their repertoire to offer the right kind of help for addiction. With the huge wealth of knowledge a GP needs to acquire and learn it is hardly surprising if addiction has not been an area covered in depth. The specialists in addiction treatment are found in Rehabs across the country. It is not the way for everyone of course and there are cost implications, but most rehabs if talked to will suggest other avenues of help. Not everyone will want to try a 12-step treatment centre but there are many that do and many who remain sober and clean because of it.

The body actually is the first area that requires attention – detoxing with medication in a safe and controlled way through a rehab is sometimes the best way of achieving the initial abstinence. Detox is the most difficult and sometimes dangerous times in the story as the body can go into extreme shock when a substance that has been used sometimes for years is stopped. The different substances have different effects and need different attention. Many addicts are fearful of the withdrawal state as it can be painful or debilitating. So detoxing with help is mostly recommended by specialists for heavy substance abuse and daily users. It can be dangerous sometimes if the body is deprived of something it has become used to it can react in confusing ways. Medical help is most definitely the preferred way of stopping. Withdrawals can be everything from sweats to shakes to hallucinations to seizures. Many peoples withdrawals are not so frightening, but some are. The length of time it takes to withdraw depends on use and length of duration and the state of the body internally as well as age. Most of the damage done in addiction cannot be seen as it is the internal organs and brain that are affected. The initial withdrawals are usually the worst, but it is important to note that there are post-acute withdrawal symptoms. This means that adverse symptoms in terms of emotions and physical problems can re-occur for up to two years after the initial stopping period.

The Body

Assuming our hapless sick addict has heard the message of abstinence and they have detoxed safely, what else needs to happen? Their nervous systems will be wired, they will be jumpy and prone to many exaggerations. Feeling sick and downhearted, again it is not unusual at this stage for an addict trying to get clean or sober to think 'if this is what recovery feels like I don't want it' The individual needs lots of re-assurance at this stage, that the way they feel is simply a stage of recovery, that they will feel better in time. Becoming newly sober or clean or stopping a behaviour that one has always turned to especially in times of stress is hard. The body can protest. What has been the go-to for years of abusive usage is suddenly it seems, stopped for no good reason other than other people wanting me to stop. (Thinking distortion)

This is where effective communication and connections come in, a partner or loved one has little understanding of what is occurring in the body of a newly sober addict and cannot even if they want to at this stage do or say much that could help. Other addicts who have traversed this place have the answers and can communicate reassurance that this is simply a stage of recovery, it is uncomfortable but will pass. For an addict though these uncomfortable times are intense, and the desire for them to end with the thing that always made them feel better and at peace with the world will be strong. It is why sometimes rehab is the best option for some, they will be looked after and the deadly substance or behaviour impossible to engage with. Let us say harder to engage with, for even in rehab the desire to use is so strong for some that even with the most stringent of checks, a substance is somehow bought and ingested, which obviously results in the person having to leave the facility. Nothing about this illness is logical. Looking at it from the outside it just looks crazy, which of course it is. The person grappling with the addiction however does not see it in the same way as non-addicts. It is a compulsion an obsession and so strong at times it breaks even the strongest willpower. In fact willpower is useless against this foe.

Other Things a Healthy Body Needs

Many addicts have serious sleep issues, some have used their substances to get to sleep. Everything about their systems are off balance, they may need medication to help in the initial stages of detox but must be cautioned that it cannot last as sleep medication is usually highly addictive. They have to be taught about **Sleep Hygiene**. Life has been anything but regular, some live the twilight life, of late nights and equally late mornings. Their body clocks are out of kilter, and insomnia when they try to change is common. To create a regular rhythm takes a bit of planning and again much reassurance from others. Melatonin is a substance created in the body and is what is needed for good sleep to happen. In addicts it is just one more of the normal bodily chemicals that does not function correctly. Doctors can sometimes prescribe melatonin, and for addicts should be tried if sleep remains elusive.

A timetable of sorts needs to be constructed to enable the individual to see what and when things need to be done. The habit of drinking **coffee** late into the day needs to change, the truth about all **stimulants and sugar** needs to be understood. The effects of all of these things on the body is profound and stopping some of them are equally profound. It is not easy to break some of these habits but important non-the-less. A regular and **nutrient rich diet** needs to be consumed. Fast food and junk food will not help the body to re-calibrate and be soothed. Most people see these initial components of a sobriety plan as sanity.

The absence of these things in life lead one to insanity. It is interesting to think of sanity in this way, sanity involves the small regular things of life that when deprived of leave a person in a fragile mental state.

There are many things that trigger a person to want to use again. These all have to be discussed, and solutions discovered. Peoples triggers are varied and personal. The taste, smell, or touch of something can be evocative to the newly sober person, people places, and things easily trigger a desire to use. Just from this one example, one can see how far a recovering person needs to go in order to stay stopped. Music for instance can be a huge trigger, and so some types of music and certainly concerts or festivals need to be stopped for a time, until the individual becomes stronger and builds a stable foundation. It is pointless to frequent venues where every person met, or every chord played leads a newly sober person to get triggered and begin to crave their drug of choice. There is no enjoyment of what can be considered an enjoyable past time only the need for the drug again. This need tends to grow and grow until it is satisfied, or something occurs to break the spell.

Triggers and Cravings

Recovering people need to learn how to manage a trigger and the craving that ensues, the cravings themselves are horrible to experience. Thinking does not enter the room; it is simply a bodily reaction with the brain opening up those neural pathways that lead to using. There are medications that can help, but again, someone with more sobriety can testify that these feelings will pass, but the experience has to be communicated about and something 'new' engaged in. If the person having a craving uses, all that happens is they enter a merry-go-round of stopping and starting with no real recovery to speak of. The act of stopping and starting is also essentially extremely dangerous to the body and does more harm to it than continued use. Nobody knows these things at the start of sobriety, they have to be communicated about, and only people who have been 'there' or work with addiction can know what they are and how to manage them. A loving partner or friend who desires sobriety for their loved one does not know this happens, so cannot advise on what to do. These states in a person's life are random and personal, to the on-looker they might look indulgent or just plain crazy. Understanding the disease of addiction is the only way to get through these initial stages of recovery.

The mind of someone who takes dangerous poisonous substances or engages in behaviours which bring disaster is not normal. The behaviour is obsessive and compulsive and in no way appears normal to the on-looker, or sometimes even to the addicts themselves. The poor mental health aspect of addiction can be seen in the decision-making process of most addicts. When eventually they are able to accept they need abstinence and are trying to remain sober the problem does not magically go away. It is not unusual however, for people to believe that all that has to happen is the using to stop. Unfortunately, the stopping part is only the beginning, and in many ways the easy bit as everyone knows what has to happen. The next stages are akin to a magical mystery tour, with good times and bad, all which have to be managed without the addiction.

The Mind

Our thoughts and dreams, our memories and experiences are all created within our mind encased in our brains.

Neuroscience has been discovering many answers that were previously hidden from doctors and scientist and of course us. We know for instance that we have intricate patterns of electrochemical pulses. When this activity stops, so do we. The activity can also change due to injury or drugs, remember alcohol is just another drug. Without an environment with emotional care the brain cannot develop normally. Trauma in its many guises affects this environment. The brain goes through impressive changes from birth and childhood to adulthood, changes that can occur in the brain can alter the fabric of who we are. It is not just illness or chemicals that change us but everything that we engage in contribute to the neural networks that makes us uniquely us. Chemical imbalances in the brain create imbalances of thinking and living, it is therefore not so hard to see that ingesting or engaging in addictive actions either substances or behaviours can lead to huge changes to what is considered 'normality'. It is this that confronts the newly sober person. Massive changes are taking place again in the brain. Unseen and not really understood. A newly sober person can feel that nothing seems right, everything is difficult or impossible to negotiate, the feeling responses to someone going through this can be seen and described as childish, with many instances of stroppy behaviour or self-pity which in children is understandable and tolerated, not so much in adults. Unreasonable behaviour comes from unreasonable thinking, so once again the newly sober individual needs others who will communicate this is just a stage and will change in time. It is this part of our human psyche that must always be catered to in a recovering person's life. We are told we should not trust our own thinking, or our minds in early recovery, are we not the people that thought it was a clever idea despite the various consequences we endured, that it would be fun to get high and we did it repeatedly. I go as far as to suggest that trusting ALL of our own thought process's years into a recovery must be treated with caution. I have made monumental mistakes based on what *I thought* was a sound decision. It is not hard to run our ideas past someone with more knowledge than us, it is not so hard to do really, yet repeatedly addicts make decisions based on their own thinking and get themselves into a crisis. The consequence of relapse is one of the things that can happen and does happen often when addicts base their lives on self-will again. The things that help in this area are:

- Abstinence from all mood-altering substances and behaviours.
- Engaging in the meetings of the 12-step movement, finding a sponsor, someone who acts as a guide. This person will discuss with us the 12-step process.
- The 12-step process is a series of tasks, if you will, that enable changes to happen in thinking and life. They cannot occur without help.
- Constructing a timetable and engaging in 'healthy' habits.
- Looking after our bodies, with diet, and sleep, regular exercise, the right medication.
- Visiting with a GP and not ignoring trivial things that are going wrong.
- Taking up some activities that promote well-being, such as yoga, meditation, mindfulness, breathing exercises, any of the eastern disciplines that will help shape and calm those neuro transmitters.

- Engaging in some mental activity that will exercise the brain. Working the 12-step programme does this for us, as we are instructed to think, be challenged, and write about self in ways that seem foreign at first. But engaging in activities, learning new things all bring satisfaction to us and are essential for a contented life.
- Engaging in therapy with trained people, either alone or with partners to challenge old ways of thinking and developing new ones. The 12-steps do some of this work but cannot do it all. Sometimes the old trauma states or issues in life need a measured and 'trained' examination to change the status quo.

None of the things discussed so far can be achieved alone, yet addicts the world over try to do it alone with the result that poor choices will lead them back to using repeatedly. Most of the way of sobriety is unfamiliar territory and new territories need guides. Changing the way our minds work is a huge task, it cannot be stressed enough that to get anywhere in this task we need other people. We need to heal the relationships we have damaged; we need to make restitution to those we have harmed; we need to find ways to live a less selfish self-absorbed way. Most of the tasks of the 12-step programme lead us to these conclusions, and the last step of the twelve asks us as we change to begin to share what we have learned with others that are still suffering.

Another shocking truth about this illness is that thousands of people are in its grips and although everything I have been talking about has been known for many years, the majority of sufferers of this illness do not have a clue as to what it is, and what to do about it if they do know. Sadly the 12-step programmes are misunderstood at best, and at worst criticised and called cults. So many people take the time to voice their opinion about the 12-step groups and decry what they achieve, it is quite remarkable. You would think that one only has to look at the success stories for there to be a softening of opinion. But not likely! What is concentrated on for some people are the relapses and the people who do not get well using it. The reasons for relapse are many, some of them already discussed. It is quite mysterious why such dislike and venom is aimed at something like the 12-step groups that at its heart only wishes for people to find recovery. Other illness do not engender such malice and yet no treatment regime for any illness has a 100% success rate. We tend to accept that quite easily with some illness's, but not with addiction, I would love to know why.

I tend to focus on the remarkable story, that the fellowship grew from just two people at its heart to one hundred, a book describing its methods was written and today this movement is in every country of the world bar one or two who do not allow it Just as they do not 'allow' drugs and alcohol. The success of this remember happened before the internet, there is no advertising and no corporate backers. Yet millions use it and have succeeded.

Some people admittedly need other methods as well as the fellowship to succeed, yet this is where AA is different to the nay-sayers, it espouses everything and excludes nothing for the sake of recovery. A meeting, a therapist or rehab, all adversaries of addiction.

The Angry Disease

There is no peace or contentment that can be found if our minds continue to jangle and be pre-occupied with anger and resentment. It is such a destructive state to remain in and the founder of the AA Programme has said,

> ***'It is the number one reason people relapse.'***
>
> ***Bill W.***

Many know the feeling; most do not know what it is, how it develops and why it has such a bad rep. It is almost a forbidden feeling. Of course it is easy-to-understand anger in its most destructive form. The vicious and destructive wars that ruin our world are the easiest place to view anger at its most destructive. Communication has ceased, and it is a question of who is the most dominant. Bombs and tanks and guns and killing are the fruits of war. But the smaller wars that rage in human beings are equally destructive. I describe us all as having a small volcano active inside of us, the layers of my volcano are laced with many frustrations and irritations that life just seems to hand out. Some small, some bigger, all have the potential to derail a fledgeling sobriety or sober life. The feeling is not the problem, it is what I do or not do with the feeling that creates the problem. As with all volcanoes the layers continue to fester, bubble away and remind us that life's a bitch sometimes. What everyone in the recovery worlds, in Rehabs, in therapists offices, and in AA rooms all know is that the layers of feeling need to be discussed. This is unbelievably difficult in the beginning of recovery as everything promotes frustration. Later on in a recovery plan the earliest memories must be searched and viewed with help.

Trauma both big and small, and most people's earliest experience of attachment are examined or should be. In many addicts these earliest experiences of life can be seen to have created some of our responses to life. The need for a substance to anesthetise life looks like a pretty understandable response to some of things people experience. Simply 'dis-ordered' attachments which can be seen in many people's lives today, and not even understood very well. Things such as an absent parent, who is away working, both care givers in jobs, problems at school. Divorce and 'blended' families. The experience does not need to be massively traumatic for the minds of some to not know how to cope or deal with life on life's terms. It is in the earliest of experiences that lead to clues for all mind detectives to find and try to bring understanding. Working out what has happened to create the response the addict has is a time consuming and laborious job. **Simply stopping the destructive substance or behaviour does nothing more than reveal what has always been the problem and what needs to be worked on and resolved if sobriety is to flourish.**

Fight/Flight/Freeze

We all most likely have heard about the fight, flight, and freeze (playing dead) response to trauma. We will have heard the terms described as our ancient survival mechanism which becomes activated when in danger or perceive danger. The feelings of either fear and or anger are the triggers to this mechanism in our bodies. A very simple explanation is the feeling activates a chemical response, usually Adrenalin, Cortisol, and other chemicals which ready our bodies for action. The process all happens in a split second with no debate or planning. Our blood pressure rises, our breathing quickens, and our hearts beat faster. The oxygen to our brain is dispersed and leaves us in the survival state of taking the action of fighting, running, or freezing. We act on instinct. This is a clever response from us as debating with the source that wants to hurt us is not a good plan. The problem in this response occurs when any unresolved trauma from our past continues to trigger the survival mechanism – PTSD – panic attacks, extreme anxiety, and depression. The original trauma can go on repeating the survival instinct in us and will go on doing so until the past can be dealt with. Just like the scratch on an old vinyl record the abnormal responses will remain until the defect can be smoothed out. Alcohol and drugs are often consumed in the mistaken belief this will help, it anesthetises temporarily, but it will continue to come back and blight a life and even make one more susceptible to anxiety until it is properly dealt with through therapy. Sometimes you will have no clue as to why the anxiety is active, but a forensic digging into past (with help) can often give explanations to what is really going on.

This work on anger and anxiety and trauma is complex and difficult, many addicts need to seek answers that they are unable to discover alone. Sometimes anger management groups are recommended. And certainly individuals are prompted to learn what they can about anger and fear and change how they deal with it through literature and others who know some answers. Silence and hiding from whatever has gone on in an individual's life does not work and never has.

Break the silence, come out of hiding. Stop blaming others and life for all the bad breaks that have led to here and now. We must understand that we personally are the creators of our own feelings and thoughts. Yes others can be and do monstrous things and need to be stopped but destroying ourselves with a substance because of the hurt and betrayal we feel is just another insane response to other insane behaviour. Communication and Connection is essential in all this work, we will never find new answers by ourselves.

Into the story of historical angers and todays frustrations must come new ways of dealing with it. If our addicts stay silent they will stay sick. They have to talk it out and find ways of understanding the story. They may need to practice calming techniques such a mindfulness, meditation, or yoga. They need to learn breathing techniques. Also the specialised techniques such as EMDR and EFT can be used to great effect with some of these historical 'stuck' issues. There are many other things that can soothe the troubled mind, but with them all comes the need to learn from others. With a new ability to discuss and learn, our once isolated sick addict begins to change, prosper, and grow. New patterns of behaviour and new responses have to be learnt, what is old and familiar can sometimes be destructive. What is new and healthy can feel impossible at first and the old ways of thinking and acting will eventually lead back to what has always been the solution, the addiction. Addicts have to change, and they need others to show them how.

With most things we need to learn, from book keeping to cooking to sewing and carpentry we have no trouble understanding that there needs to be an apprenticeship, and in this phase of learning other people need to be consulted who pass on their knowledge. It is the same for most things we need to learn, so in this most complex of illness's with the most tricky of rules for recovery it is no different. Why on earth do people persist in believing they can do it by themselves? - Makes no sense. - But as we are discovering not much makes sense in the active stage of addiction – Remember simply stopping the using behaviour is only one part of what needs to occur – The brains and minds of addicts continue to make poor decisions based on self-will. For the addict, lives based on self-will are doomed to failure, and doomed to make the same mistakes again and again.

EMDR:
Eye Movement, Desentisization and Reprocessing

EFT:
Emotional Freedom Technique

Each is a therapeutic technique which aids in dealing with trauma and other emotional disregulation.

6:

Self Esteem

What is eroded so often in an addicts life, as they traverse the progressive journey into addiction is this thing we call self-esteem. Perhaps as children there were incidences which also eroded confidence and esteem. Things such as trauma, big and small, disorganised care giving, or attachments all play a part in shaping a person's response to life. If a mind-altering chemical is introduced into the mix it is not too hard a leap to see the outcomes may not be good with or without early trauma.

Our addicts may have started using simply because it is the fastest way to gain confidence in social situations, addiction takes shy nervy people and turns them into party people. Shy and nervy are the usual feelings for most teens, with them not really realising it. This added to the sensory augmentation of most addicts, creates the perfect reason to use and continue to use. This only ensures our shy nervy teen never learns how to deal with things like social situations, as it is the drug or addiction that is in control. Self-esteem and confidence grows usually as we grow and mature, but addicts get left behind in these areas.

As the addiction progresses then the behaviour also deteriorates, with any value system that may have been in place also being shot to pieces which ensures that self-esteem and confidence remain in very short supply.

At the start of any recovery an examination of the behaviour when using has to take place. It is not unusual for the person trying to get well to feel everything from shame and disgust about what they have become, to hopelessness and despair that it is too late for change to make any difference, and that their families would be better off without them. It is not rocket science to discover that all of these feelings do not a good recovery make. They have to be talked about, worked on, and healed. It takes much work talking to therapists and other recovering people before any semblance of understanding can be felt. Some addicts have done shocking things whilst under the influence and to come out from under the blanket of despair when they are exposed is hard. One of the most healing of things could be when our addicts realise that the shame they feel may indeed indicate that some of their value systems have been broken. They actually have some - just broken! Most think they are just bad, or wicked and it takes a lot of convincing that what is in play is one of symptoms of the illness, and that they feel bad because somewhere inside they know what they have done is to breaks all their ideas about moral conduct. Values such as authenticity, compassion, fairness, faithfulness, kindness, honesty, and freedom all become compromised when in the grips of addiction. Confidence and self-esteem could never be in plentiful supply when abhorrent behaviours wipe out everything one really believe in.

But amends can be made, behaviour can be changed. Restitution in many forms can also be made, but our stumbling fumbling addict can never find the way into any of these solutions by him/herself. That is just impossible. Do you see how important communication and connection is? To be a person of integrity, to gain back self-esteem and worth, one needs to be engaging in estimable things. The how and the what in trying to begin all this is where other people come in. The mind, the body and the soul are all engaged in this piece of repair work.

'Be Impeccable with your word.'
From The Four Agreements
Don Miguel Ruiz

As the repair to the addicts souls, their bodies and their self-esteem begins, they are a group of people who feel extremely fragile and vulnerable. They behave anything but. Their shame may make them aggressive or continue to hide. They have to be coaxed out of hiding. They definitely need help, where else but from some of the wise souls who have gone before. Other addicts, therapist, and specialists in recovery and addiction and of course literature which can describe the healing process. In the marvellous little book described above, Don Miguel Ruiz describes a process that begins with something that most everyone when counselled about, can actually do, being honest and truthful and taking care about what comes out of one's mouth. Bill W. the founder of the 12-step programme stated, ***'honesty is a pre-requisite to recovery'.*** He of course was talking about the cessation of fighting about what is really wrong, an admittance that the substance is a problem and the need to stop. The need for honesty follows the programme endlessly. There can be no recovery without it. Don Miguel Ruiz just describes the process a little more poetically. We know our words can create beauty but also destroy it. Words uttered in anger or thoughtlessness can maim and hurt. Addicts have often not been aware of things said or done and denial is the hiding place of lies. Denial is in-grained in a practicing addict that it is sometimes impossible not to continue to lie. Careless untruths can create trauma of course and as addicts themselves are usually adorned with trauma it is the very thing that continues the destructive shame and blame game. Self-rejection is rife in the early days of someone trying to get sober. The protection of denial has been broken and the huge mess that is revealed almost appears to be impossible to heal. How can addicts have any esteem if this were to continue? Of course they could not. This is the hard work of a recovery programme. The using stops and immediately the damaged view of self is revealed. Very few addicts are proud of themselves when they first come into recovery. It has to be worked for, and behaviours, attitudes and feelings have to change. To have self-esteem, they need to be able to do things they can be proud of. Stopping the using and staying clean and sober is the first of many things that can elevate esteem to a less painful place. Repairing the damaged self needs care and meticulous work. Again this would be an impossibility if the addict were to try this by themselves. Those in the programme who have gone before and remain clean and sober, stand as clear tangible signs that it is all plausible and possible. Self-esteem is fragile in early recovery, another sign that remaining connected and able to communicate is a good idea. Perhaps it will always be a fragile thing. Becoming the 'better versions of ourselves' is the work of recovery and recovery is a never-ending project.

Suicidal Ideation

Untangling all the mysteries and complexities of the addicted individuals mind is the job of psychiatrists, doctors, and therapists and all the medical world. The fact that fragile deranged minds exist is not the prerogative of just addicts of course. But the fact that many addicts reach a place of darkness and fear and end up believing the world would be better off without them in it, is a stark fact of untreated addiction for some. Many who come into treatment and begin to talk about how they feel recognise this place of despair and shame. It is hard to talk about of course. The taking of one's own life, not so long ago, was seen as a crime, which chased the act or even thinking of the act into dark caves of silence and secrecy. But even if the fear of punishment were not the factor in keeping silent, then somewhere inside of us all we know, just know that self-destruction is going against the laws of creation. We enter the world screaming for air, warmth, sustenance, and love, what is it that changes this instinct and drive for life?

Our lives can be described as being made up of small and big traumas. Some we manage, some we don't, some are so dark we struggle to live with them. Trauma as discussed has vibrations that tangle up our thinking process's, this coupled with behaviours powered by addiction further mess with our minds. As the disease progresses, well so does the damage done to an already fragile mind and brain. Massive neurochemical imbalances dance in the dark and nobody actually can discern this unless honest communication is entered into. Something is going terribly wrong in the thoughts processes of people. Addiction brings with it at times an altered state of consciousness, so does trauma, so does suicidal ideation. This is not a healthy state, nor a rational state, nor a sane state of mind. It is often not seen and understood either by anyone close to the individual We all have the ability to wear masks and hide the truth from self and others. When you know a bit about the mind, and addiction it is not hard to understand that suicidal ideation fits into a bracket of surrender of the spirit or loss of motivation or the will to carry on living.

Other events that create trauma: foetal trauma, birth trauma, loss of parent (s), sibling rivalry, constant moving, school bullies, poverty, lack in any area of life, not being good looking enough, being too good looking, weight issues, body image, illnesses and accident, abuse of all kinds, physical, sexual, and emotional, violence, surgery and medical experience, disasters such as fire, flood earthquakes, war. In other words just about everything! Some people can deal with some of these naturally as they mature others cannot, and will struggle with life, themselves and need help.

The long-term effects of trauma and out of control addiction are alarming, debilitating and very strange. If we can view this as energy that becomes trapped in the nervous system. It perfectly describes the process where trauma cannot be resolved, and it goes on to wreak havoc inside of us. This can be clearly understood when we talk about PTSD. A fragile state of mind that remains stuck in a moment of time, constantly re-living and experiencing whatever has been lived. It is usually dramatic and frightening. The drama and the fear just play over and over in a loop, like a scratch on a vinyl record. As already described the scratch will remain and ruin the song or music until the scratch can be dealt with. Unexplored or unresolved traumas or addictions will create damage to the individual until it is dealt with. As with most mental health issues the solution we have is talking therapies, sometimes medications, often both. One thing is clear though in order to heal from any kind of trauma or addictions or to stop suicidal ideation, communication has to be entered into with someone who has answers different to self.

K. Hough
Addict

So why am I writing this? I guess it's because I'm sitting here reflecting on the news that one of my friends has just killed himself because of this cruel disease. I'm definitely feeling numb; but also can identify it is making me feel really thankful that I am still here. In addition to this I've got the opportunity to change the path of my destructive addictive lifestyle. This is why I felt so strongly that I needed to contribute to this book, because it means so much to me to try to stop this happening to anyone else.

I'm sat here taking stock of my life; in reality asking myself what actually happened? So far, I've lost my job, health, my self-respect, lost contact with my brother, and those personal relationships that I still have are very strained.

I would like to talk about what happens from my perspective, and how those important connections in my life slowly break down and disappear. My brains wiring has become twisted with this disease, so I don't often realise what I am doing to myself, my family and friends and my entire support network.

When I'm deep in my addiction nothing matters. I don't care about anything; friends, family, work, personal care, my possessions, and the list goes on. It is like I've sealed myself in a bubble. This leads to me breaking contact with everyone because I am so ashamed of what I am doing and yet continue to do it. The disease progresses, meaning that I slowly continue to disconnect myself from the world. Family and friends continue to be desperately concerned about my well-being. Slowly and surely my bubble gets smaller and smaller, and the daylight turns to darkness. I'm then existing in a black and white world where I just can't see any escape.

On top of it – I am so fed up and ashamed of telling people I have relapsed again - I remember sadly the memory of my birthday this year where I just couldn't stop crying. This was driven by feeling incredibly sorry for myself, feeling desperately alone, feeling empty and useless – in summary hating myself. I remember walking around preparing to kill myself so I could leave everything neat and tidy for my family.

It has taken me awhile to write this because I'm pausing and remembering that this disease has already claimed five years of my life. Wasted shameful time but for me this is a small price to pay compared to those that have lost their lives.

My place in rehab is booked, I am determined to get well this time and stick to the programme. I refuse to waste any more of my life.

If you bring forth that which is within you,
Then that which is within you
Will be your solution.
If you do not bring forth that which is within you,
Then that which is within you
Will destroy you.

- *from the Gnostic Gospels - Waking the Tiger*
Peter A Levine

7:

Our Souls / Our Spirits

Oh my goodness what on earth does this mean? Easy to suppose when soul-talk is engaged in that we assume that this talk about a 12-step programme and recovery, has all been a huge confidence trick and it is about religion after all. However nothing could be further from the truth. Somewhere in the literature of Alcoholics Anonymous, and in the knowledge of many who have found recovery, is the talk about what ails the addict, and it is a disease of the mind the body and the spirit. The mind and body are not too difficult to talk about and understand, much is written about each, much is known about each. The spirit however, what is that, and how do we talk about that? Some addicts are terrified of contemplating spirit/soul. It is as if the addict life precludes the experience of peace and love, which are spiritual concepts. Again the knowledge that addicts are sick people who will recover and not 'bad' who will become 'good' needs to be understood. The disease concept is truly the first understanding amongst many that has to be gained. But what has spirit-talk to do with anything, what is spirit what is soul?

A way to understand perhaps is to see that our soul houses that spirit within that glow and vibrates with life and love or shrivels and grows dim with wrong living and poison soaking throughout the body. It is the part of self that when nourished can accomplish marvellous things. Our soul is unique to each of us, and we are all able to be in touch with it. How many times have you felt shivers run up and down your spine when something beautiful is heard, seen, or discussed? How many times does the instinctual self within warn of danger? What is it that impels us to seek peace, hope, and love, to want to give this to others? What is it in certain people that destroy peace and hope?

The soul part of the human being is where it all gets interesting when we try to discuss it. In one of the steps of the programme we are asked to 'make a decision to turn our will and our lives over to whatever we consider is the power greater than self'. If we are able to remain sober by following the directions of others that we meet in our recovery then this has already happened. We are then invited at this stage to think about the bigger questions of life such as 'who am I' or the meaning of life and talk about the soul fits neatly into these discussions.

We know intuitively that soul has to do with honesty, realness, and depth. These aspects of our humaneness that become depleted when in the grips of an addiction. Nothing grows well, it is gloomy and lonely. We are of the world, but not really. Our minds gripped with a thousand problems, none of them enlightening or beautiful. We dare not imagine soul and spirit as we know we are damned. It is after all a disease of mind, body, and spirit.

Tenzin Gyatso
Fourteenth Dalai Lama of Tibet (1936)

I call the high and light aspects of my being spirit and the dark and heavy aspects soul.

Soul is at home in the deep, shaded valleys. Heavy torpid flowers saturated with black grow there. The rivers flow like warm syrup. They empty into huge oceans of soul.

Spirit is a land of high jewel-like lakes and flowers. Life is sparse and sounds travel great distances.

There is soul music, soul food and soul love.

People need to climb the mountain not simply because it is there but because the soulful divinity needs to be mated with the spirit.

- from The Soul of the World,
Cousineau/Lawton A Book by Harper Collins

The Disease of More

In the grips of any addiction, by its very nature the addict continues to want more, and however much is used it is never enough. I visualise those neural pathways of the brain with small grasping hands, demanding, imploring, beseeching more, more. I need it want it and must have it, and it must be NOW. That craving and that obsession is exceptionally demanding. As I observe it now from the safety of sobriety, I can see it was demanding my life and with it my soul.

We strive to be sated, satisfied by buying, owning, having endless things, supposing they will make us happy, the most fabulous of relationships, the next new car, a stunning home, diamonds, and pearls, - well you get the picture – Something 'out there' is what we need and will fill this emptiness I feel. For a while it works, but the shine wears off the new possession, and a good relationship takes challenging work and attention, the diamonds and pearls are pretty but kind of useless, someone will always have something bigger, better more impressive than we have.

Strange then to think that a beautiful poem, the scent of a flower, the kindness of strangers, or a stunning piece of art in one of the great museums, or a successful sobriety, can fill us with the type of feeling we are always searching for. This feeling cannot be bought or owned; it is bestowed on us if we are lucky. If we do experience it, naturally we want to keep it and keep it shiny and glowing, however as it is not a 'thing' it cannot be seen, owned or bought. It can be worked on though and again the answers to how, can be found in the 12-step programme and sobriety.

Addicts must stop doing the very thing that kills their souls. They achieve abstinence.

They find others that can help them find answers and learn to trust them rather than their own thinking. They have to be able to understand that their best thinking got them to the place they currently are, and if that is in a fellowship meeting or rehab, they have to be able to see their thinking must have been going terribly wrong for some time.

They clean house, which means they start to unearth all the parts of their personality that no longer serve them well, if they ever did, and work on changing. Again this change that needs to take place cannot be achieved alone.

The change in their personality starts a process of seeing the world differently, they no longer want so much, or demand they are right, they open up their minds, accept that there are some things that cannot change. They are able to find their humanity and make restitution for the things done wrong. They are forgiven and can also forgive. To be able to let go of years of shame and sorrow is the most amazing thing. It creates a lightness in being, which invites all addicts to discover more.

In this process they are able to glimpse parts of the soul, they realise they are not bad people, but have been blind and sick. They begin to discover who they really are, who they really should have been before addiction took them down to slavery and despair, and it is the release from these prisons that allow their spirit to come alive.

In the work addicts have to engage in to keep sobriety they learn about spiritual matters. They read literature by some of the amazing minds in the world. They look at different religions to try to understand what compels a person to choose whatever path they have. They try different things and in the trying of many things that are available to us in our world they eventually find their own true path. What they should be doing with the life they have left. When this occurs and is cherished and looked after, a sense of gratitude begins to emanate. The power then to help or benefit others will be found and in this behaviour is an immense satisfaction. In recovery one can move from selfish, self-seeking behaviour into people that can truly discern that life should be more than the desire to own or possess things or people. Freedom is found and that soul thing that was incomprehensible becomes something that is just known.

In his interesting book 'Care of the Soul,' Thomas More writes:

A soulful personality is complicated, multifaceted, and shaped by both pain and pleasure, success, and failure. Life lived soulfully is not without its moments of darkness and periods of foolishness.

I love this description because it speaks of the journey of recovery, which is not all plain sailing. Things tried sometimes fail, people loved turn out to be the wrong fit, the experience of losing a loved one to death is unbelievably painful and distressing. These things are what shape us and define us. To know the pain means we can empathise, to fail at one thing makes us try harder with the next and be grateful when we succeed. For addicts negotiating all the pitfalls of life without the enveloping arms of the addiction is a feat in itself. However if it is accomplished the resulting refining of self becomes open to soul work.

None of the things talked about can be accomplished alone or in solitude. Addicts do not turn into pious people living lives of retreat and prayer. Instead they have to interact first with the people who can help, from the meetings or therapy that they choose to engage in, and then with the wider world.

The point of all the work done on self within fellowship and therapy rooms is to unearth the best version of self. This task is impossible for anyone if people are clothed in layers of trauma sadness and shame. We all have to be taught how to disrobe. How to view life experiences differently. How to let go, how to forgive self and others and how to accept. Little words, 'let go, forgiveness, and acceptance' but so difficult to achieve sometimes.

Acceptance Forgiveness and Letting Go

Years of selfish self-seeking behaviour that was in control when in the throes of addiction is a hard almost impossible task for the newly sober person to change. They have to understand how to achieve it in the very first instances of a recovery programme, they have to accept they are sick people, they have to accept they have an illness, and have to accept they need help to deal with it. A very tall order, but if they do it, they are 'gifted' with the ability to achieve abstinence.

However this is not the only time they are instructed that acceptance is one of the keys to serenity and/or sobriety.

If our addict continues to live a life with unexplored issues that they are unable to deal with, things from childhood, disordered attachments, trauma big or small, events in life that leave them perplexed and hurting they will not remain sober for long even if they can find it in the first place. The addiction after all is the solace for whatever ails their spirit.

If they are able to be honest with someone who possesses some different answers to any that they have been able to find, and they are able to do some of the suggested things to heal and grow it means they have accepted something outside of self which will help them They communicate with *this other* and in this process find some connection. These things do not always happen with everyone we meet. However if they can trust one other person and in that trust begin to work on things that have blighted life, they are able to enter a different way of doing things. Eventually discovering they cannot travel far if consumed with rage, fear, or resentment. They have to understand these are blocks to the way forward. Forgiving self happens first through understanding that good people can do unbelievably dreadful things under the influence of mood-altering anaesthetic like substances, that thinking has become very distorted in the pursuit of any addiction, that what ails addicts is an illness that was not their fault in the first place.

This is so liberating and if believed can be the start of forgiving self. If self can be forgiven, than the next task is to forgive others. A seemingly impossible task at first, but with diligence and honesty and a whole lot of understanding and love the way through can be found. Once understanding that forgiveness of others does nothing for those being forgiven, but everything for the one forgiving. It helps to disentangle self from the twisted thinking and all-consuming hatred, fear, or anger that is felt. The release of these feelings are the gift of forgiveness.

It does not mean we absolve others for their part in our pain, but we resist the urge for vengeance and in so doing free self from their influence. In the focus we have for vengeance anger or resentment we allow the other to have power over us. It is the feeding ground of addiction. Forgiveness frees and releases us.

If this happens we have learnt how to 'Let Go'. If this is achieved, it makes room for new experiences. In letting go we change the direction of our thinking; it frees up space and sets the scene for new more beneficial things to nourish and benefit life. This is the healing process that began with the first tentative acceptance of the fact that to move forward abstinence needs to be gained.

Addicts discover in sobriety that this acceptance, forgiveness and letting go process is something that has to continue throughout life if they hope to retain sobriety. It is what impels addicts to remain connected and communicating with others who walk the same path as them.

Bill W. one of the founders of the 12-step programme is quoted as saying in one of his books, The AA way of Life - 1967 AA World Services:

'We are not cured of alcoholism. What we really have is a daily reprieve contingent on the maintenance of our spiritual condition.'

There is no spiritual condition with a heart full of hurt rage or fear. These conditions of course can be present with or without addiction and can come and go according to the events in our lives. They are not dispelled simply by not drinking or drugging or engaging in the addiction of choice. The absence of the chemical or addictive behaviour is simply what enables us to really 'see' and gives us the ability to find the solution. After all if the euphoric wrappings of addiction are what can soothe us then why the need for all this arduous work? However one simple truth about recovery and the millions of people who now embrace it is that *being soothed* by the addiction was not how it remained. No-one comes seeking support or help from a rehab, therapist, or fellowship meeting because life is fabulous. Trouble, shame, despair, and hopelessness are the companions of addicts at the start of any recovery journey.

Sobriety is a state of mind, not only the absence of the things that make up addiction.

Relapse prevention is at the heart of everything that is done to manage addiction. Paying attention to mind, body and soul are the essential components to walking the journey to a better version of self and a better life.

Insanity?

What exactly is insanity?

A definition of this word in a dictionary is: 'mentally deranged' but what does that mean? We all experience reality differently, and we experience reality through our sensory perceptions. Our eyes do not really see, sound is not taking place in the ears, touch is not really happening in our fingers, and smell not with our nose although they all feel as though the experience is in seeing with our eyes, ears touch etcetera. However they are not direct senses, they are all taking place within the control centre of the brain, yet the brain has no direct access to the world, so it is our sensory organs, eyes, ears, nose, mouth, and skin that function as interpreters.

How amazing is that?

The information is gathered from many sources and is translated into the common currency of the brain. The electrochemical signals of our marvellous brains. There are many hundreds and thousands of electrochemical signals and pulses sending messages every second of life. Every sight, sound, smell, and touch rather than being direct experience is an electrochemical song played in a dark and mysterious chamber. Vision, smell, sound, and touch feels so effortless, yet the brain exerts enormous effort to construct these things. Understanding and reality emerge from the interactions of all the data collected from each sense. Every night in sleep we enter a sensory deprivation chamber yet can continue to have intense and colourful dreams or even horrifying nightmares. We know what is real and what is dream state when we awake. We also know what things are. The knowing comes from comparing information from things the brain has already constructed, its updated, refined and corrected continuously and we do not even realise it is going on. A marvellous high-tech computer really. Sci-fi like in its execution – it is no wonder sci-fi is such a popular genre, we recognise something that is mysterious perhaps?

It is not hard to understand reading all of the things just written that if these processes are corrupted in some way and chemical imbalances occur we can experience delusion. So many mental health illnesses can be understood in this way. Something goes wrong with the processes of the brain.

Insanity then is also something that has gone wrong in the brain.

Observe a drunk person, how they speak, how they walk. Can they safely drive that car? Can you always tell when they are in blackout? What is going on in a brain that has been anesthetised?

Observe someone who has had lines of coke, or any of the pills and potions that addicts turn to, are they mentally competent? What creates the insatiable need of increasingly more of whatever drug is being ingested. Are their electrochemical neurons working correctly?

Observe a habitual gambler, spinning his or her life away at the roll of a dice or the colour of a card.

Observe a sex addict, changing partners often, desperate to feel sated and then this satisfaction that can only be found in the next person, and the next, and the next.

What goes on in these brains and minds? What drives that often-incomprehensible behaviour in addicts?

Observe a depressed person, an anxious person, a person with ADHD, a person with suicidal ideology.

All brain states that can be described as not normal.

The dictionary definition talks about insanity as being mentally deranged. I would state that all the examples above could be viewed this way. Yet this is not quite how we understand insanity. What we tend to think about insanity is when the person hears voices or obeys voices other than their own or does things because the voices instructed them to. Or a person who does things mostly outside of the norm, and lacks insight. We tend to think of dark and dangerous individuals and incomprehensible actions as being insanity. In court, a prisoner who is deemed insane has done things outside of normal awareness and who lacks insight, and they are often cruel and mystifying things to everyone else. We 'normal' people have nightmares about them!

Perhaps it is easier to think about what is sanity? It is an interesting question as most people I have ever asked the question talk about things that are so terrifyingly normal, like eating and sleeping and getting up at regular times. Having a job and a life to be proud about. By abstinence, once realisation that addiction is the problem, by being kind and honest and true to others. By talking and loving and staying in the 'normal' realms of life. So if this is what sanity is, than insanity is the absence of these things, and in advanced addiction of course these are the very things that are in short supply.

It is the actions that perpetuate these states that are in the behaviour of every addict. They become progressively worse over time. The disease is progressive.

One can only surmise that the electromagnetic neurons, the neural pathways that are being created in severe addiction are created by brains that are deranged. Therefore can be viewed as illness, and maybe even insanity.

Have we reached an understanding of insanity?

Maybe, in some people's minds addiction cannot be seen as an illness because it is 'self-inflicted,' the psychopath was born that way – Humm - there are most definitely research papers published that discuss the genetic precursors that help create an addict. These are present at birth, are not ordered, or chosen, or anything, they just are: they need certain actions by the person to activate them, and it is this that most people who view this illness as self-inflicted see. Yet many people experiment or try various mind-altering things in the growing up process and not everyone activates the addiction gene. So perhaps it is this that gives addiction is disturbing stigmatization?

Certainly, some addicts do cruel and vile things whilst under the influence, but addict's do not automatically resort to the same pattern of behaviour. The urge to hurt, kill or abuse is abnormal, and something that exists in some, not in others. There is definitely a 'derangement' in someone who exhibits these things. Psychopathy has books devoted to it. The neural pathways created in addiction are different and whilst 'under the influence' a person may act deranged, but there is a difference between addiction and psychopaths.

I continue to ponder and puzzle about the stigmatization of some mental health illnesses, as some are definitely viewed differently. Take suicidal ideation for instance it has only fairly recently lost its 'criminal' status. Yes it used to be against the law to kill oneself, even though most of us can view a mental state such as personal destruction as not being in any way something a person with normal functioning would choose. It was the fear of punishment or being stopped forcefully that drove suicidal ideation into such a secretive state. Happily, these days there is a more gentle view of this sad state of mind. In that gentleness maybe we can find more ways to stop people destroying themselves, and certainly more people may be willing to stop hiding the thinking. Making it easier then to do things to help.

It is actually also what could change the dreadful statistics of death by addiction. So many people are on the road to self-destruction with the illness of addiction, yet the majority of the time it is seen as a selfish, self-inflicted thing, even by addicts themselves, many do not know they have an illness because it is not how the majority view it in the world. So addiction hides behind denial, secrecy, and silence.

For treatment to work, what needs to happen is for the individual to be able to experience reality, look at his or her own behaviour with others that do not judge or condemn. Take a look at what has been going on and be given choices about what to do about it. If the person does not wish to change, then nothing will change, and the illness will continue in the individual destroying every aspect of life. This is the stark fact about addiction unless change happens it continues until one is destroyed.

Mark Murphy one of my dear friends, wrote the next poignant piece as he was going crazy on his boat alone in Amsterdam just before he made it into treatment for the second time, Christmas 2018. He is a musician, and poet, an ex-therapist and sailor of the seven seas. He is marvellous and clever, talented, and lost his way despite knowing so much about the programme. As the poem clearly states it was lack of communication and lost connection that led to a frightening state of mind. He often talks about this period being one of the worst bouts of insanity that re-occurred after several years in the programme. What led to this, is his story, but he has kindly allowed me to share this piece in the book.

"Over here!"
"Hey,
Can't you hear us from there?
We're dying trying to get you back involved
but it's tragic
Seeing you so distracted by your usual day today
Plans and thoughts we heard you say would
kill you
Not one of us disagreed
Having severed so much connection
Your magic retwists into insanity"

M. Murphy 4/12/2018
Fisher Lady/Amsterdam

8:

Relapse

The relapse rates in this illness are huge. So frequent that it leads some people to think there is simply nothing to be done about any addiction. This however is simply not true. There are many addicted people who have discovered a way to live free from addiction, and relapse. Many people who continue to remain sober and have never relapsed. To discover more of how to do this, it is important to understand something called Post-Acute Withdrawal, PAW's for short, as well as looking at some of the stages of relapse. Each have a potent message to impart which could function as an early warning system and in so doing save anyone from an actual devastating relapse itself. Perhaps also knowing that relapse can happen anytime be it 6 days, 6 weeks, 6 months or 6 years – there is no time limit in this illness. If one fails to pay attention to recovery the illness strikes.

Post-Acute Withdrawal (PAWS)

Most people understand and know about withdrawal symptoms, if not experienced personally than we have seen movies where the addict attempting to get clean is depicted going through a painful experience, things such as the sweats, and shakes, cramps, or any number of uncomfortable experiences also sometimes very scary things such as hallucinations, paranoia and fits or seizures. These things are usually well known and feared sometimes by addicts who have relapsed and know they must go through it again. These are the body and brain trying to re-calibrate and rid the system of the poisons it has been ingesting sometimes for years. What is not known however is that some of the psychological symptoms can re-occur for anything up to two years. Again as the brain functions and chemistry try to return to a normal state. Things such as mood swings, depression, tiredness and irritability, low energy levels and a depleted sense of motivation, which can all be part of the initial withdrawals. The symptoms are not felt by everyone, but in those that do experience them they report they can come and go with no warning. What needs to be remembered with these symptoms is that they are temporary and will eventually change and stop. As long as the person going through them does not give up, feeling that sobriety is not worth it if this is how they must live. Again it is the brain and body trying to heal and our addicts must be told it will not last forever. The way through this assault on the body and brain can only be traversed with communication and connection, someone to tell the addict 'Its ok, you will not die, it will not last forever,' can make all the difference. We are encouraged to do 'nice' things for self, talk and do not be alone. Step up therapy or meetings, just do not return to the thing that has created this in the first place. Having a holistic view of what needs to change about how we have lived is important, a regular timetable, practicing sleep hygiene, healthy food, and nutrition, not too many stimulating foods and beverages, watch the sugar intake. Its normal living really, but remember addicts rarely live 'a normal life'. Adjusting and living life on life's terms tends to be met with a whole lot of difficulty, and certainly our apprentice recovering addict needs much encouragement to keep going. Because for all the ailments felt the addict knows the thing that will sort it out quickly and return them to euphoria. Their addiction of choice. In these moments, the reality of what will actually transpire is lost to the addict who is not in reality. Their electrochemical synapses are firing around like pinball machines.

If they are aware of these symptoms and know what to do about them they will then be better prepared to recognise them when activated and do the things to survive.

The Three Stages of Relapse

Relapse prevention needs to be etched into the psyche of recovering people. Relapse prevention should be in everything they do. Some things that they think or do will take them closer to a relapse and some things they think and do will protect them from relapse. Figuring out what these things are should be recovery's number one priority. There are distinct stages that could be warning signs if taken notice of. They can be broken down into issues in the mind, physical signs then the actions that lead up to the relapse.

Emotional Relapse

At this stage, most addicts are not thinking about using. But some emotions and behaviours could be setting them up to relapse in the future. Some of the signs of emotional relapse are, anxiety, anger, intolerance, mood swings, isolation, not asking for help, not going to meetings and poor eating, and sleeping habits. In fact all the behaviours and feelings our addict has tried so hard to alter from the start of recovery, at this stage if they recognise the position they are in as serious and do something about it they can still pull back from relapse. This needs to be taught, it is not automatically known.

Mental Relapse

At this stage they have some kind of war going on in the mind. There are some desires to use, but they know they should not. It is just day dreaming or toying with the notion. Some of the signs will be, thinking about the people they used with, places and things involved in using remembered as fun and exciting. Glamourising it all. Lying. Hanging out with the people who they used to have such fun with. Planning how and when they are going to use. At this stage they are in fantasy land, none of the thinking is truth.

Addicts have to do things like **play the whole tape**, see what happened on a regular basis when they started to use before, disaster and hopelessness usually.

Tell someone what is going on in their heads.

Use distraction techniques. Call a friend, go for a walk, anything to change the way the thinking is lying to them.

Physical Relapse

Once the relapse thinking starts something has to be done about it. Addicts cannot push the thoughts away as they will become more insistent. They also cannot successfully block out the thoughts. A programme really has to kick in to help if the thoughts are there otherwise the actual physical using is a heartbeat away. It is hard to stop the process at this stage, and addicts need to take notice and act long before they get to the point that they are driving to see their dealers, or going to the pub.

Hopefully by now you can see that just stopping the active using is just a tiny part of what has to happen to effect a successful recovery. Without abstinence of course addicts will achieve very little, but IF ONLY abstinence is achieved then recovery will become de-railed very quickly. If addicts stay isolated, they will be de-railed. If they fail to make the right connections they will become de-railed. It is actually quite a simple equation but so very difficult to do first of all and then to keep on doing.

Why should this be such an obstacle for so many people?

It can only be because addiction is such a mis-understood illness. The fact that the thinking process is severely flawed is rarely considered, and truly it is hard to accept, especially if in some other areas of life they are successful. Addiction can only exist if the denial systems are in place. It is this process that pushes the addict into secrecy and lies and a desire to hide the truth even from themselves. The other very important consideration of course is that the addict knows the using has to stop and as the most prominent thought process for most addicts is the obsession to use. Addicts are all in a no-win situation. The only way out is education, knowledge and understanding. It is what makes the anonymous fellowships so powerful, here the misunderstood, the sick and the frightened will find understanding and in the sobriety of others realise that recovery is possible.

More Warning Signs That Could Lead to Relapse

Dishonesty

This creates such an easy route back to using. Patterns of little lies and secrets create mayhem in the mind. Remembering who, and what lie was used to whom and when is exhausting. Equally damning are the lies told to self, rationalising occurs as addicts make excuses for not doing what they should or doing what they should not.

Impatience

Things are not happening fast enough, or others are not behaving how you want them to. Every little thing just scrapes on the brain like chalk on a board. Nothing feels right any more, and the tension is growing.

Controlling Behaviour

Destructive in all sorts of ways. Mainly it takes the emphasis off of self and focuses on others. This is no way to heal yourself. But if I focus on your faults and failings and try to dictate what you should do there is less chance that my failings will stand out.

Omnipotence

You now have all the answers for self and others, no-one is able to tell you anything and you even ignore suggestions from others. You forget the mess life has been running on self-will.

Argumentative

You argue about small inconsequential things, this goes with the previous heading. The need to be right is strong. Self-will is in control.

Frustration

If things do not go your way you blame others, it actually makes you their victim, but this is not seen at the time. The feeling if not checked continues to grow.

Self-Pity

An ugly sad feeling to drown in, 'why does this always happen to me, why do I have to be an addict?' 'It's not fair' are usual refrains.

Unreasonable Expectations

I have changed why can't they? You have not yet seen the work that needs to happen to encourage healing in others. They need to see your commitment before anything else. Yet unreasonable behaviour blinds you to this truth.

Lack of Gratitude

All of the above suggestions have a lack of gratitude in their appearance in your life. You must find some again and quickly. There is no gratitude to be found in any relapse. It is also said that grateful people will never relapse.

To become strategic in the avoidance of relapse is important. Remembering that we are also dealing with the Glutamate (memory) component of addiction, means we should:

- Prepare for triggers.
- Avoid triggers as much as possible, risky people and

risky places. But remembering that music, smells, certain films and definitely people can always prove triggering.

- Healthy self-talk in moments of craving – play the whole tape.
- Certain medications can help or hinder, become aware.
- Get to meetings, have a network of help

For some the damage done to the brain is massive and sometimes cravings and drug seeking becomes unconscious, more automatic like driving your car at times without really thinking about it. Or being vaguely aware that what was being done (around drugs and alcohol) was none too smart. Or there I was again with a drink in my hand thinking this time things would be different.

With continued drug use and withdrawal another system is recruited by the brain to counterbalance excess dopamine. Our hedonic setpoint (pleasure setpoints) revert to allostasis which is a change of the hedonic setpoint under stress in an attempt to maintain stability. This results in anhedonia – an inability to find pleasure in normal pleasurable activities. Most addicts end up in this state, those patients that enter treatment can nearly always be observed as taking a long time to revert to normality. The sadness and low moods are not always due to the consequences of drugged actions but down to the brain not functioning normally Pleasure or contentment is in short supply, this state lasts for weeks sometimes. It takes hard work to construct a workable living regime and a life that creates pleasure and satisfaction. There is a lot that can sabotage even the strongest of will power.

Hormonal Imbalances

Hormonal dysregulation is another serious area which cause some to relapse and relapse and relapse and not know why. For some the agony of going through a regular monthly torture trap is now being recognised as something that can destroy peace of mind and also recovery. The hormone dysregulation cause the feelings and thoughts of people trying to stay clean and sober to go into a spin, with dark terrifying thoughts and behaviours which look insane and to those who suffer this certainly feel insane. Escape into a drug of abuse is sometimes the solution and the ever-increasing nightmare. Alcohol and drugs become the medicine that is sought. It brings temporary relief, which unfortunately does not last. The monthly cycle is sometimes difficult for many, but PMS, PMT, Menopause, Post Natal Depression and other symptoms associated with hormonal cycles are all states where everything is magnified and exaggerated, the person feels in a whirlwind of black emotion. The substance is the answer and the problem again as it does nothing but increase the madness that the hormonal eruptions are causing. In my experience this is an under developed area of medicine. We advise seeing the specialists in this area of medicine. Gynaecologists who specialise in hormonal dysregulation and menopausal problems are the people with the answers for this particular nightmare.

9:

Re-building Our Lives

In the re-building of life that addicts all have to become involved in they have to engage in many things that previously they gave little thought to. Once abstinence has been achieved and our addict begins to feel better, it is easy for them to think that is all that needs to happen. However this first phase of re-building is only the beginning. The relief and joy many addicts feel when the first few months of clean time are experienced and the pats on the backs and relief of partners and friends, can lead to everyone thinking that this is it, we have done what needs to be done and all is good. This is sometimes known as the honeymoon period or a pink cloud fantasy, and it is what the terms suggests, **not based on reality.** Addicts tend to have a black and white view of life, they need actually to learn how to navigate the grey, the middle ground. This is unfamiliar territory for them and will need patience, understanding and a whole lot of help. Getting through all the hurdles of early recovery alone or isolated will not work. Those recovery connections that have to be made are the people who can help with this. A family member or friend will have no clue that the addict has more he needs to learn, and many addicts who mistake the honeymoon period for how life will always feel, are often ambushed by reality. When the pink cloud disappears, and the grey appears it is only another addict or someone who knows about the recovery process that can tell everyone how to change the grey.

The self-esteem of a newly recovered person will be fragile, the thinking will still be prone to exaggeration and the propensity to dramatize events will be strong. Learning how to negotiate all of these pitfalls is hard but necessary. Confidence and self-worth which is lost in the progression of the illness can only begin to repair if abstinence and a determination to change is agreed upon. For some the sober vistas of life are too difficult to negotiate without the substance, but the substance and addiction continues to destroy everything until it is stopped. This is the truth about this illness. Calling it an illness is often thought of as a 'cop out' and all the person has to do is stop, 'just say no' goes the famous Nancy Regan quote. Yet stopping without some of the knowledge that has been talked about in these pages cannot happen, the addicted person does not know they are ill, and that abstinence is only one of the keys needed. They cannot possibly understand what goes on in the neural pathways of their brains, so unless they talk to people, stop the using and begin to work for change they are destined to just become worse and worse until they die.

Perhaps if they had said no before any substance or behaviour was engaged in - maybe. However, at the time of the first drink drug or addictive behaviour they see 'everybody' else doing this and they do not want to seem different. It feels so good too, the euphoric high is quite seductive and the 'feel good' part of the illness serves to entice them to use and use again. After all is it not woven into the fabric of modern life? A drink or two calms any amount of stress, is the thing that makes a party swing and life more joyous. Only a percentage of our happy party goers have the addictive gene and brains that go bonkers when substances and addiction take over. Most people who are addicted do not even know it until disaster becomes part of the story and is endlessly repeated. The story of addiction is complex, confusing and continues to baffle everyone. Re-building self and life after years of acting in a destructive self-seeking way takes time, patience and connection with others who can tell the addict what needs to be done and what needs to be continued to do.

Abstinence from ALL mood-altering chemicals, now and always.

Finding a support network of other people who understand and support recovery.

Changing old habits, staying away from risky people places and things.

Investing with time and sometimes money to learn more about what goes wrong in addiction. Therapy perhaps, definitely literature and DVD's.

Creating a workable timetable to keep on the straight and narrow.

Understand that 'the narrow' will only feel this way at the start of the journey.

Do things that calm and soothe the mind. Things like yoga, mindfulness, meditation and breathing exercises. Doing things we thought were only for other people to do. Explore and discover. Embrace silence.

Silence is so hard to obtain, silencing the addict's mind enables them to hear and 'know' what needs to be done to get well.

Calming the body enables addicts to experience the 'now' and begin to hear.

Working with others to understand the traits and

behaviours that drive the addiction.

Make amends to people that may have been harmed. Telling them the truth and not expecting anything in return.

Continue to delve into new thinking and beliefs, discovering worlds that were previously hidden.

Attempting to be the best version of self and to try to help others find some of the answers that have helped in this quest.

So, the very many and varied things addicts need to do to stay well begin with abstinence, communication, and connection. Re-building a life free from addiction takes time and patience and lots of help. It also takes persistence. Relapses are part of the story of recovery for some people. Relapse every time it occurs is like seismic shudders that wreak more havoc in the body and brain of people who really should not experience any more damage. The fact that a relapse can occur at any time, six days, six weeks sixteen months even sixteen years and all the numbers in-between, after a life has been rebuilt is another strange phenomenon in the addiction world. Relapse can occur and re-occur at any time in the addicts life. It is one more warning sign that addicts need to remain connected to the knowledge that got them clean and sober in the first place. It's a lifelong job to care for the crazy brain that is hardwired to want to do things or take substances that end up destroying them.

I am better now.

Maybe one will not hurt?

I can control it.

Surely after all this time it must mean that perhaps I was

not really an addict in the first place?

I cannot possibly need to continue to do all the things I needed to do when I first got sober.

Surely going to a bar, or a casino or a festival cannot hurt?

I am bored doing the same thing repeatedly, I want some fun.

Life is dull, no sunshine, no excitement.

The obsession of every addict is to be able to use again normally, and the most insane thing any addict can do after a period of clean time is to use.

That story is a never ending one, it is told in the various recovery rooms up and down the country. No-one who has relapsed ever comes back to tell a great story of how wonderful the drink or drug was or how much they enjoyed their latest losses at the casino. Every person who makes it back to a recovery room after a relapse tells the same heart-breaking tale of shame and destruction. It is bizarre listening to these stories as they all start sounding like the same refrain. "I stopped going to meetings, I got bored with the programme, I thought I was better now, I wanted some fun." Whatever the motive was to use again, what becomes crystal clear is that the flawed thinking that started this mess in the first place was in control. This is so visible to everyone except the addict. The only way to keep this piece of knowledge visible is to stay connected to a recovery programme. The only way to access any recovery programme is to communicate with people who frequent the recovery rooms.

Admittedly this sounds a bit freaky, a bit like a secret society, a bit like an exclusive club, which of course it is. Its exclusivity remains because no-one who does not have this illness would be seen going to a place like a recovery meeting, even addicts still get shy and secretive in the beginning. Sadly, the stigmatization of this illness is strong and continues unabated. The way addicts think and behave is different when in the throes of whatever addiction is running the show. The fact that the brain of an addict performs differently even in recovery is sometimes a fact that is missed or mis-understood. The defect in the brain that constitutes flawed thinking is a lifelong issue, which will require lifelong attention to keep it managed. In times of high stress or distress the addict needs to know their brains are creating environments where the easiest thing in the world is to return to the thing that has always offered the most comfort and promise of pleasure. Addicts have to work hard to find those things in different ways. Taking a substance is easy and quick, the other ways are hard and never quick.

Children – Part 2

The discussion about children is so important, they are our next generation of either brilliant and happy adults or the opposite, likely to develop addictions of their own or other mental health issues.

Most of the parents who have come into treatment for alcoholism sincerely believe that they have successfully hidden the worst or all of their drinking/drugging from their children. This is not so. Little children are curious and interested usually in anything parents do. They are curious and notice behaviours, but they are terrible interpreters, they do not understand the finer details of course. Older children copy friends and are influenced by what their social groups do, so attitudes to alcohol and drugs need to be discussed at home It is reported that by the age of five a child who has watched a parent drink has already formed opinions about alcohol. They will ask questions but if one tries to dissuade them from knowing about alcohol because they are 'too young,' their curiosity will know no bounds. Explaining to them that their little bodies cannot tolerate, or digest alcohol is a good start. If children live in households where out of control addiction is present then they see, hear and experience things they should not. They understand alcohol makes daddy angry, or mummy sad. I have heard stories of children pouring alcohol away to 'protect' their parent. They may be aware of the arguments and out of control behaviour, they grow up traumatised sometimes by things never meant to be directed at them. They also become the targets at times of the 'grownups' whose semblance of humanity is being drained by their use of alcohol or drugs. Children will pick up and 'eat' pills and potions, will notice powders left lying around. Children have died because of it. Of course these are extreme examples of what can happen, but most definitely the next generation of addicts are in the 'training ground' Sensible drinking rules and the dangers of taking drugs should be a conversation at home, impossible whilst all sensibilities are in trouble in the parents behaviour. There are organisations that have been formed to help young kids deal with their own addictions, as getting hooked early is not an impossibility. All families should become alcohol and drug aware, if children don't encounter it at home they will encounter it in their social circles. This scourge (addiction) to modern life is absolutely everywhere!

Disease or selfish choice?

So to all those who doubt that addiction is an illness, or that it is a cop-out to call it a disease, or think addicts choose to be so self-absorbed in active addiction. What you need is the information of just what it takes to remain clean and sober when one has the disease. It has never been a question of just saying no. If this were the case there would be no relapses, as anyone who has an addiction and used a programme to get better, knows all the information that is told in these pages, it is what recovery and treatment are all about, disseminating this knowledge to those who need it.

Why would they use again if the very fact that their knowledge of the programme means they had to find it from a position of destruction, fear, and pain? The insanity of the destructive part of addiction is that the walls of denial and not seeing are strong, the ignorance that surrounds recovery is epic. Believing that recovery will work if all that is done is to stop the using persists. Hardly anyone non addict knows the defective brain stuff, and even some addicts dispute it, yet does it not make the most perfect of sense? What else could possibly explain the madness we see in practicing addicts. Returning to active using is easy. Remaining connected and continuing to communicate saves addicts from making terrible mistakes and believing that 'one won't hurt, or I'm better now,' The defective thinking is in charge and at fault, if all this could be known, and society were to call addiction a mental health issue with addicts who have brains that create flawed thinking. If this were universally accepted, then those dreadful statistics of death by addiction would fall. It is time to change, to be a kinder more wise society. One person at a time, one day at a time it can happen.

We have only this moment, sparkling like a star in our hand – and melting like a snowflake..

Sir Francis Bacon 1561 – 1626

Resources

Alcoholics Anonymous – World Service –
www.alcoholics-anonymous.org

Pleasure Unwoven – DVD – Kevin Macauley
www.instituteforaddictionstudy.com

National Association for children of alcoholics NACOA

Narcotics Anonymous world Service inc.
www.na.org

The Four Agreements – Don Miguel Ruiz
ISBN 9780880889902

The Soul of the World – Cousineau/Lawton
ISBN 0062510045

The Brain – David Eagleman
ISBN9781782116615

The AA Way of Life – a reader by Bill
AA world service inc.

Care of the Soul – Thomas Moore
ISBN 0749911689

Waking the Tiger – Peter A. Levine
ISBN 9781556432330

Chasing The Scream – Johann Hari
ISBN 9781526608369

I Blame the Hormones – Caroline Church
ISBN 9781909771307

One Breath at a Time – Kevin Griffin
ISBN 1579549055

Nicabm – www.nicabm.com
(National Institute for the Clinical Application of Behavioural Medicine)

Al-Anon and Families Anonymous - The fellowship as a whole for developing, growing, and including many more Anonymous meetings for all the numerous addictions that are in our world today.

Acknowledgements

I continue to acknowledge the huge service Bill W and Bob made to my life and the millions that follow the 12-step programmes. Without them I may not have lived to discover the life I have today.

Steve Stevens who helped me see my 'truth'

Grateful thanks for their personal and ongoing support by submitting extracts to give this book the human realness that it has, you are all much admired.

Dr Simon Kelly – Consultant Psychiatrist
MBBS MS (Psych) FRC Psych

Angie Cullen – RMN – Family Specialist
Addiction Therapist

Anne Barton
Secondary School head teacher and Leadership consultant

Libby Garnham
Founder, Chairperson of ANA Treatment Centre

David Musgrove – Managing Director

Mark Murphy – Musician, poet, ex-therapist, and sailor.

Lloyd Haylor-Smith – Trainee Addiction Therapist

K. Hough – Addict

A thousand thanks to Angie and Libby for once again assisting me in editing and checking facts. You are brilliant.

If you have enjoyed this book or

Found it helpful…

Please leave a review on Amazon

The mission is to

'Change perceptions one book at a time'

Please join me in this quest.

www.sarinawheatman.com

Also by Sarina Wheatman

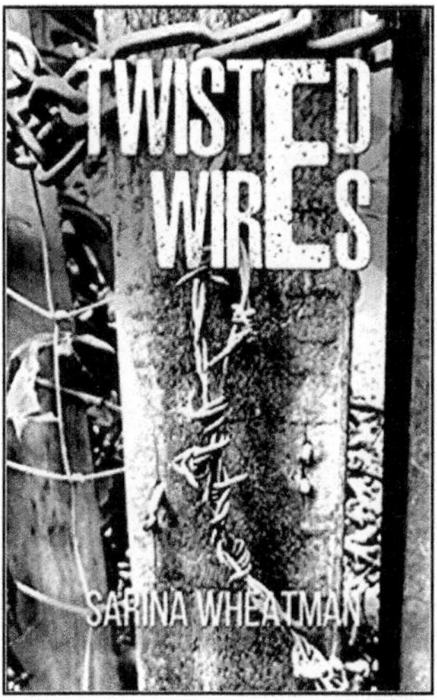

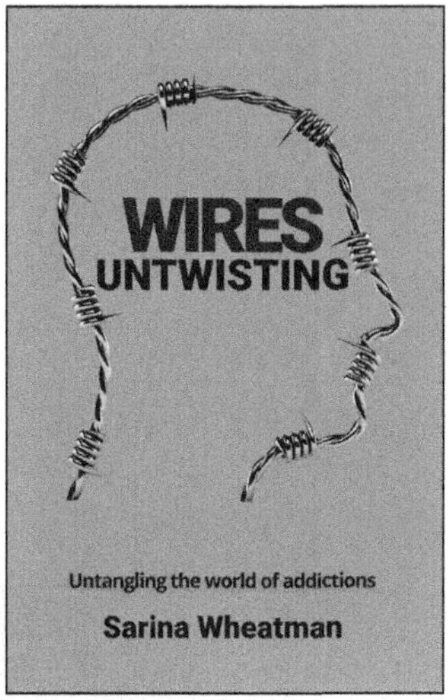

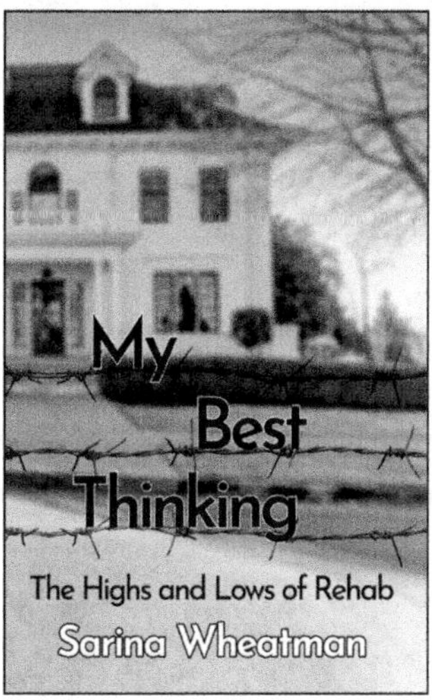

Available worldwide from Amazon

---

www.mtp.agency

www.facebook.com/mtp.agency

@mtp_agency

Printed in Great Britain
by Amazon

84409934R00089